AF750423

YOUNG ADULTS WITH SERIOUS MENTAL ILLNESS

YOUNG ADULTS WITH SERIOUS MENTAL ILLNESS

DAVID O. SULLIVAN
EDITOR

Nova Science Publishers, Inc.
New York

For permission to use material from this book please contact us:
Telephone 631-231-7269; Fax 631-231-8175
Web Site: http://www.novapublishers.com

LIBRARY OF CONGRESS CATALOGING-IN-PUBLICATION DATA

Available upon request

ISBN: 978-1-60692-641-3

Published by Nova Science Publishers, Inc. ✢ New York

CONTENTS

PREFACE

The transition to adulthood can be difficult for young adults who suffer from a serious mental illness, such as schizophrenia or bipolar disorder. When these individuals are unsuccessful, the result can be economic hardship, social isolation, and in some cases suicide, all of which can pose substantial costs to society.

Due to concerns about young adults with serious mental illness transitioning into adulthood, this book provides information on (1) the number of these young adults and their demographic characteristics, (2) the challenges they face, (3) how selected states assist them, and (4) how the federal government supports states in serving these young adults and coordinates programs that can assist them.

In: Young Adults with Serious Mental Illness
Editor: David O. Sullivan
ISBN: 978-1-60692-641-3
2009 Nova Science Publishers, Inc.

WHAT GAO FOUND

GAO estimates that at least 2.4 million young adults aged 18 through 26—or 6.5 percent of the non-institutionalized young adults in that age range— had a serious mental illness in 2006, and they had lower levels of education on average than other young adults. The actual number is likely to be higher than 2.4 million because homeless, institutionalized, and incarcerated persons were not included in this estimate—groups with potentially high rates of mental illness. Among those with serious mental illness, nearly 90 percent had more than one mental disorder, and they had significantly lower rates of high school graduation and postsecondary education. GAO also found that about 186,000 young adults received SSA disability benefits in 2006 because of a mental illness that prevented them from engaging in substantial, gainful activity.

Young adults with serious mental illness can have difficulty finding services that aid in the transition to adulthood, according to researchers, public officials, and mental health advocates. Because available mental health, employment, and housing services are not always suited for young adults with mental illness, these individuals may not opt to receive these services. They also can find it difficult to qualify for adult programs that provide or pay for mental health services, disrupting the continuity of their treatment. Finally, navigating multiple discrete programs that address varied needs can be particularly challenging for them and their families.

The four states GAO visited help young adults with serious mental illness transition into adulthood by offering programs that provide multidimensional services intended to be age and developmentally appropriate. These programs integrate mental health treatment with employment and other supports. To deliver these services, states use various strategies. They coordinate across multiple state agencies, leverage federal and state funding sources, and involve young adults and their families in developing policies and aligning supports.

The needs of young adults with serious mental illness have also received attention from the federal government, and agencies have been providing some support to states through demonstrations, technical assistance, and research. Federal agencies have also established bodies to coordinate programs to serve those with mental health needs, youth with disabilities, and youth in transition, which may help improve service delivery for young adults with serious mental illness, as well.

WHY GAO DID THIS STUDY

The transition to adulthood can be difficult for young adults who suffer from a serious mental illness, such as schizophrenia or bipolar disorder. When these individuals are unsuccessful, the result can be economic hardship, social isolation, and in some cases suicide, all of which can pose substantial costs to society.

Due to concerns about young adults with serious mental illness transitioning into adulthood, GAO was asked to provide information on (1) the number of these young adults and their demographic characteristics, (2) the challenges they face, (3) how selected states assist them, and (4) how the federal government supports states in serving these young adults and coordinates programs that can assist them.To do this work, GAO analyzed data based on national surveys, including the National Comorbidity Survey Replication (NCS-R), and administrative data from the Social Security Administration (SSA). GAO also reviewed published research; interviewed federal, state, and local officials, as well as mental health providers, experts, and advocacy groups; and conducted site visits in Connecticut, Maryland, Massachusetts, and Mississippi — four states that focus on this population.

GAO did not make any recommendations. HHS made comments intended to clarify the report and we made changes as appropriate.

ABBREVIATIONS

CMS	Centers for Medicare & Medicaid Services
CPS	Current Population Survey
DI	Disability Insurance

DOD	Department of Defense
DOJ	Department of Justice
DOT	Department of Transportation
DSM-IV	Diagnostic and Statistical Manual of Mental Disorders–Fourth Edition
HHS	Department of Health and Human Services
HUD	Department of Housing and Urban Development
IEP	individualized education program
NBS	National Beneficiary Survey
NCS-R	National Comorbidity Survey Replication
NIMH	National Institute of Mental Health
SAMHSA	Substance Abuse and Mental Health Services Administration
SSA	Social Security Administration
SSI	Supplemental Security Income
TIP	Transition to Independence Process
TRF	Ticket Research File
USDA	U.S. Department of Agriculture
VA	Veterans Administration
WIA	Workforce Investment Act

June 23, 2008
The Honorable Pete Stark
Chairman
Subcommittee on Health
Committee on Ways and Means
House of Representatives

The Honorable Gordon Smith Ranking Member
Special Committee on Aging United States Senate

The transition from adolescence to adulthood is a challenging time in which individuals assume greater responsibility for their independence and make critical decisions about relationships and careers that affect them long into the future. While this transition can be difficult for all young adults, it is particularly so for those who suffer from a serious mental illness, such as acute schizophrenia or acute bipolar disorder. The interpersonal skills and sound judgment most needed during young adulthood are precisely those skills that can be impaired by a serious mental illness. Moreover, the severity of mental illness can vary over time, and experiencing severe episodes during this transition period can derail young adults from completing school or beginning a career. When young people with serious mental illness do not successfully transition to adulthood, the result can be economic hardship, social isolation, and in some cases suicide, all of which can pose substantial costs to society.

While public mental health services are primarily administered by states, a variety of federal programs can assist young adults with serious mental illness as they transition to adulthood. Because of concerns about young adults with serious mental illness transitioning into adulthood, you asked us to provide information on (1) the number of young adults with serious mental illness and their demographic characteristics, (2) the challenges they face, (3) how selected states assist these young adults, and (4) how the federal government supports states in serving these young adults and coordinates federal programs that can assist them.

To provide information on the number and demographic characteristics of young adults, which we define as individuals aged 18 through 26, with serious mental illness,[1] we analyzed data from two surveys of individuals living in U.S. households: the National Comorbidity Survey Replication, 2001-2003 (NCS-R), a federally funded survey of mental illness, and the Census Bureau's 2006 Current Population Survey, Annual Social and Economic Supplement (CPS). We estimated the prevalence of serious mental illness using the NCS-R, which is based on interviews conducted from 2001 through 2003. We then applied that prevalence estimate to the number of young adults aged 18 to 26 nationally in 2006, as estimated by the CPS, based on the assumption that rates of mental illness were relatively stable in this age group between 2001 and 2006. We also analyzed two Social Security Administration (SSA) datasets on individuals receiving disability benefits: the 2006 Ticket Research File (TRF) and the National Beneficiary Survey, 2004 (NBS).[2] We assessed the reliability of data from the NCS-R, the CPS, and SSA and determined they were sufficiently reliable for the purposes of this report. We also reviewed published research on the extent of mental illness among the homeless and those involved with the criminal justice or foster care systems.

To identify the challenges faced by young adults with serious mental illness, we reviewed published research as identified through a literature review of relevant journals, books, articles, and reports published since 1995. We also interviewed federal, state, and local officials during site visits to four states (see below), mental health providers, and experts in the field of transitional young adults and mental health. Finally, we interviewed advocacy groups, as identified throughout our review, that work with young adults and their caregivers.

To describe how selected states are assisting young adults with serious mental illness, we visited four states that have implemented programs specifically focused on this population: Connecticut, Maryland, Massachusetts, and Mississippi.[3] During the site visits, we met with officials from mental health agencies, other state agencies, private organizations involved in providing or advocating for services for this population, and, when possible, young adult consumers of mental health services. We selected these four states for our site visits because, after reviewing published research and interviewing federal and state officials, mental health researchers, and advocacy groups, we determined that they offered statewide or state-organized programs specifically focused on transition-aged youth with serious mental illness.[4]

To determine how federal agencies are supporting states and coordinating federal programs that can assist young adults with serious mental illness, we interviewed federal officials from agencies within the U.S. Department of Education (Education), Department of Health and Human Services (HHS), Department of Housing and Urban Development (HUD), Department of Justice (DOJ), Department of Labor (Labor), and SSA. We also reviewed documents pertaining to the activities and accomplishments of interagency coordination groups as well as funding and eligibility information on federal programs relevant to young adults with serious mental illness. See appendix I for a more detailed description of our methodology. We conducted our work from June 2007 through June 2008 in accordance with generally accepted government auditing standards.

In: Young Adults with Serious Mental Illness
Editor: David O. Sullivan
ISBN: 978-1-60692-641-3

Chapter 1

RESULTS IN BRIEF*

We estimate that at least 2.4 million young adults aged 18 through 26—or 6.5 percent of the 37 million non-institutionalized young adults in that age range—had a serious mental illness in 2006, and they had lower levels of education on average than other young adults. This estimate of 2.4 million is likely to be low because certain groups that may have high rates of mental illness, such as the institutionalized, were not included in the NCSR. Nearly 90 percent of young adults with serious mental illness had more than one type of disorder. For example, 32 percent of these young adults had a drug or alcohol-related disorder in addition to another type of mental disorder. We also found that, compared to young adults with no mental illness, those with serious mental illness have significantly lower rates of high school graduation (64 versus 83 percent) and continuation into postsecondary education (32 versus 51 percent). Our analysis of SSA data indicates that, in 2006, about 186,000 young adults with serious mental illness received disability benefits because their mental illness was determined to be severe enough to prevent them from engaging in substantial employment. We were unable to identify the number of young adults with serious mental illness who were homeless or involved in the justice or foster care systems; however, evidence suggests that young adults in these groups have high rates of mental illness overall.

Young adults with serious mental illness face several challenges, including finding services tailored to their specific needs, qualifying for adult programs that provide access to mental health services, and navigating multiple programs and delivery systems. Existing public mental health, employment, and housing

* This is an edited, excerpted and augmented edition from a United States Government Accountability Office Report GAO-08-678, dated June 2008.

programs are not necessarily tailored to their mental disability or age range, which may discourage these young adults from participating. For example, officials in three states we visited stated that Workforce Investment Act (WIA) youth centers could not provide the intense, customized support that young adults with serious mental illness need, and state officials also indicated that there are not enough permanent housing options tailored to this age group. With regard to access to mental health services, those who received free or low-cost services as children may not qualify for them as adults. According to the National Council on State Legislatures, states' clinical criteria for receiving public mental health services are generally narrower for adults than for children. Similarly, Medicaid income requirements are more stringent for adults, and differences in criteria for child and adult disability benefits from SSA can result in a loss of benefits during redetermination at age 18 for youth who had received benefits as children. Finally, researchers and public officials cite the difficulty young adults with serious mental illness may have navigating the multiple discrete programs that may address their varied needs.

The four states we visited—Connecticut, Maryland, Massachusetts, and Mississippi—have developed programs that offer multidimensional services designed for young adults with serious mental illness as they transition into adulthood. The services are intended to be age-appropriate and to address various needs, such as mental health care, vocational rehabilitation, employment, life-skills development, and, in some cases, housing. In Connecticut, the program initially focused on individuals referred from the Department of Children and Families, but it has since evolved to focus on a broader group of young adults with serious mental illness. This focus is similar to that of the other states' programs. The state programs vary in size, with some serving a relatively small number of young adults, and none have been systematically evaluated to determine their effectiveness. States have used a variety of strategies to provide these services to young adults with serious mental illness. One strategy has been to coordinate services across multiple state agencies by establishing formal referral processes or launching interagency task forces. This strategy can provide a bridge for individuals who were receiving services and supports from one agency as children and must transition to another agency in order to continue to receive those services and supports as adults. Another is to leverage resources by combining funds from federal and state sources. States have also used certain service delivery models promoted by the Substance Abuse and Mental Health Services Administration (SAMHSA) as evidence-based practices. One such practice, supported employment, assists young adults with obtaining and retaining competitive employment in the community as part of their mental health treatment. Another strategy has been to involve young adults with serious mental illness and their family members in developing policies and aligning services for these programs.

The needs of young adults with serious mental illness have also received some attention from the federal government, which has, to some extent, supported state efforts to serve these young adults and is beginning to coordinate programs that can assist them. While we found that there are currently no federal programs that specifically target this population, SAMHSA and Education formerly sponsored the Partnerships for Youth in Transition program of 2002-2006 to foster state-funded programs for transition-age youth with serious mental illness. This initiative has yielded ongoing collaborative transition programs at several sites in five states: Maine, Minnesota, Pennsylvania, Utah, and Washington. An evaluation of the young adults participating in the programs suggests that there may be some positive outcomes for them, and SAMHSA plans to promote similar initiatives in other states. Federal agencies also fund other demonstration projects that support state and local efforts to provide or better coordinate existing services for transition-aged individuals, although these programs are not targeted to young adults who have a serious mental illness. In addition, federal agencies are providing some support to states and localities through technical assistance and research. For example, Labor's National Collaborative on Workforce and Disability for Youth provides technical assistance to One-Stop Centers to increase their capacity to serve individuals aged 14 through 25 who have disabilities, which include serious mental illness. Additionally, the National Institute of Mental Health (NIMH) is funding research on innovative strategies to better serve this population. In response to presidential concern about uncoordinated service delivery in the mental health and other related systems, several federal agencies have formed working groups to consider opportunities for collaboration among programs that involve mental health, youth in transition, or the needs of transitional youth with disabilities, although none are focused on young adults with serious mental illness.

We provided a draft of this report to Education, DOJ, HHS, HUD, Labor, and SSA as well as draft sections concerning their states to Connecticut, Maryland, Massachusetts, and Mississippi. We received technical comments from all of the federal agencies and states, which we incorporated where appropriate, and general comments from HHS. In its general comments, HHS indicated that the report was pertinent and timely but expressed some confusion over our definition of serious mental illness and noted that the report's scope could be expanded in a number of ways. We clarified our definitions and noted that, while additional research could be beneficial, the scope of our report focused on the objectives and population agreed upon with our requesters. Written comments from HHS are included in appendix VIII.

In: Young Adults with Serious Mental Illness	ISBN: 978-1-60692-641-3
Editor: David O. Sullivan

Chapter 2

BACKGROUND

Young adulthood is a critical time in human development. During this period, individuals transition into roles that they maintain long into the future. This transition can involve completing school; securing full-time employment; becoming financially independent; establishing a residence; entering into a stable, long-term relationship; and becoming a parent. To successfully accomplish these things, young adults must develop good interpersonal skills, sound judgment, and a sense of personal responsibility and purpose.

The transition from child to adult roles can be a challenging one, and evidence suggests that this period has become longer and more complex over the years. During the 1950s, young people often completed their education and secured employment, married, and became parents all in their early 20s. Since then, the economy has grown increasingly information-driven, while wages have declined and the cost of living has increased, when adjusted for inflation. Consequently, young adults require greater technical skills and education to support themselves and may alternate living in an educational setting, with their families, or independently well into their adult years.

MENTAL ILLNESS AND DISABILITY

As they transition to adulthood, some young people may experience a mental illness, which is generally defined as a health condition that changes a person's thinking, feelings, or behavior and causes the person distress and difficulty in functioning.[5] Some young adults develop their mental illness during childhood, while it is typical for others, such as individuals with schizophrenia, to experience the onset of symptoms as young adults.[6] Although research shows that 50 percent of mental disorders begin by age 14,[7] it can take several years for the illness to be detected and appropriately treated. Early detection and treatment of mental disorders can result in a substantially shorter and less disabling course of mental illness.

The symptoms associated with a given type of mental illness can vary in frequency and severity across individuals and for each individual over time. Mental illnesses with particularly severe symptoms can have a dramatic impact on an individual's ability to function in everyday life. The fatigue experienced by an individual with major depressive disorder can be so severe that it is difficult to summon the energy to work every day. The delusions associated with paranoid schizophrenia can make it impossible to maintain stable personal relationships with spouses, coworkers, or friends. Certain other mental illnesses are known for the unpredictable and episodic nature of their symptoms and the harmful effect this has on the ability to function consistently over time. For example, individuals with bipolar disorder can alternate between periods of mania, relative normalcy, and profound depression. For a young adult, such unpredictable mood swings can stymie progress in securing and maintaining a job or beginning and sustaining a long-term relationship.

Individuals with mental illnesses who have particularly severe symptoms can qualify for certain federal supports. The Alcohol, Drug Abuse, and Mental Health Administration Reorganization Act of 1992 uses the term serious mental illness to identify individuals whom states are allowed to treat using federal dollars from the Community Mental Health Block Grant program.[8] In response to the requirements of this Act that HHS develop a definition, SAMHSA defined "adults with a serious mental illness" as those who are: "age 18 and over, who currently or at any time during the past year, have had a diagnosable mental, behavioral, or emotional disorder of sufficient duration to meet diagnostic criteria specified within DSM-III-R, that has resulted in functional impairment which substantially interferes with or limits one or more major life activities." [9] These major life activities can be basic living skills, such as eating or bathing; instrumental living skills, such as maintaining a household; or functioning in social, family, or vocational/educational contexts. States are free to establish more restrictive eligibility guidelines for their treatment population in several ways: by narrowing the list of qualifying diagnoses, specifying the length of time the individual must have had symptoms, or requiring that individuals function below a certain level. As a result, the criteria used by states to qualify adults for public mental health services can vary.

Some individuals with a serious mental illness may be unable to work because of their impairments. These individuals aged 18 or older may qualify for Supplemental Security Income (SSI) or Disability Insurance (DI) provided by SSA if they can demonstrate that their mental illness results in the inability to engage in any kind of substantial gainful activity and has lasted or can be expected to last at least 12 months.[10] DI pays benefits related to prior earnings to those with a work history sufficient to obtain insured status. Children can receive DI benefits based on their parent's work history.[11] SSI provides cash benefits for those who have limited or no work history and whose income and assets fall below certain levels. Children can receive SSI benefits if they have a qualifying disability themselves. Individuals may receive concurrent payments from both DI and SSI if their work history qualified them to receive DI payments but their income and assets—including the amount of their DI payments— were sufficiently low that they also qualified to receive SSI payments. In fiscal year 2006, approximately 8.6 million individuals received DI payments and 6.9 million received SSI payments, for a total of $126.4 billion in benefits paid out over the course of the year.

PUBLIC MENTAL HEALTH SYSTEM

Many people with serious mental illness receive treatment through the public mental health system, which serves as a safety net for those who are poor or uninsured or whose private insurance benefits run out in the course of their illness. State mental health departments have primary responsibility for administering the public mental health system. In doing so, they serve multiple roles, including purchaser, regulator, manager, and, at times, provider of mental health services. Services are delivered by state-operated or county-operated facilities, nonprofit organizations, and other private providers. The sources and amounts of the public funds that mental health departments administer vary from state to state but usually include state general revenues and funds from Medicaid and other federal programs.

The services provided by the public mental health system to individuals with serious mental illness have changed over time. Historically, state-run public mental health hospitals were the principal treatment option available to them. By the 1960s the reliance on inpatient care was viewed as ineffective and inadequate because of patient overcrowding, staff shortages, and other factors. At the same time, improved medications were reducing some of the symptoms of mental illness and increasing the potential for more individuals to live successfully in the community. A recovery-oriented, community-based approach to mental health treatment has since emerged. Under this approach, individuals are to receive services and supports uniquely designed to help them manage their mental illness and to maximize their potential to live independently in the community. These services and supports are to be multidimensional— intended to address not only mental illness but also employment, housing, and other issues. When feasible, these multidimensional services are provided in what is referred to as a "wrap-around" manner—that is, they are uniquely targeted to the nature and extent of each individual's needs. When services are provided by multiple agencies, those agencies are to coordinate their activities and funding so that the individual experiences the services and supports seamlessly—as if from one system, not many.

Federal Programs that Can Assist Young Adults with Serious Mental Illness

Services and supports relevant to young adults with serious mental illness that are funded or provided by federal programs include mental health treatment, education and employment assistance, housing, and income support. In all, the Judge David L. Bazelon Center for Mental Health Law (Bazelon) identified 57 relevant programs in 2005. (See app. II.) These programs are administered by a variety of agencies, including DOJ, HHS, Education, HUD, Labor, SSA, and U.S. Department of Agriculture (USDA).

Programs Funding Mental Health Services

The federal government funds mental health services that are provided by programs administered by state agencies. Table 1 lists five examples of such programs.

In particular, Medicaid and the Community Mental Health Block Grants are major sources of federal funding for mental health services for young adults with serious mental illness. Medicaid is a health insurance program for certain groups of low-income individuals, including elderly and disabled individuals and children.[12] Funded jointly by the federal government and the states, and administered federally by the Centers for Medicare & Medicaid Services (CMS),

Table 1. Examples of Federal Programs That Can Provide or Fund Mental Health Services to Young Adults with Serious Mental Illness

Department	Program	Purpose
HHS	Community Alternatives to Psychiatric Residential Treatment Facilities Demonstration Grants Program	Five-year demonstrations to help provide alternatives to psychiatric residential treatment facilities for children up to age 21 and allow coverage of a comprehensive package of community-based services for these youths such as 24-hour support and crisis intervention, respite care for families and after-school support programs
	Community Mental Health Services Block Grant Program	Provide mental health services to people with serious mental illness
	Comprehensive Community Mental Health Services for Children with Serious Emotional Disturbances	Promote more effective ways to organize, coordinate, and deliver mental health services and supports for youth up to age 22 and their families
	Medicaid—Medical Assistance Program, Title XIX	Improve access to health care for low-income individuals and those in certain groups
	Projects for Assistance in Transition from Homelessness	Provide mental health and related services to homeless individuals with a serious mental illness

Source: GAO analysis.

Medicaid is the primary federal payer for public mental health services provided by states. In order to receive federal Medicaid funding, states are required to provide certain broad categories of services, such as inpatient and outpatient hospital services and physician care. Reflecting their medical focus, Medicaid mental health services have traditionally been provided by physicians, including psychiatrists, who work at hospitals, clinics, and other institutions. While Medicaid will cover services provided to individuals in facilities with 16 or fewer beds, the program specifically excludes coverage provided in large state-run psychiatric institutions for adults aged 22 through 64. States may choose to provide certain optional categories of services. For example, states may use the Medicaid "rehabilitation option" to cover a broad range of services related to rehabilitation from a mental illness or other condition or disability.[13] States may also participate in certain Medicaid demonstration programs that allow them greater flexibility in the services they choose to cover. Medicaid spending by the federal government and the states totaled $317 billion in 2006.

To supplement the Medicaid program, CMS administers several smaller grant programs that states can use to fund improvements to their mental health systems. For example, CMS established Medicaid Infrastructure Grants to support state efforts to enhance employment options for people with serious mental illness and other disabilities. States may use these grants to plan and manage improvements to Medicaid eligibility determination and service delivery systems or to improve coordination between the state Medicaid program and employment-related service agencies. Nearly $43 million was available to states under this grant program in fiscal year 2008. CMS also administers Real Choice Systems Change Grants to help states and others build the infrastructure that will result in improvements in community-integrated services and long-term care supports for individuals with long-term illnesses and disabilities, such as serious mental illness. The goal of the program is to help these individuals live in the most integrated community setting suited to their needs, have meaningful choices about their living arrangements, and exercise more control over their services. Nearly $14 million was awarded to states under this grant program in fiscal year 2007.

Through the Community Mental Health Services Block Grant program and other federal grant programs, SAMHSA funds mental health services that can be used by states to assist young adults with serious mental illness. The block grants are allocated to states according to a statutory formula that takes into account each state's taxable resources, personal income, population, and service costs. In order to receive the funding, states are required by SAMHSA to provide data on the mental health services provided including demographic information annually to SAMHSA on the number of individuals treated by the state's mental health system. In addition, states are required to maintain statewide planning councils that include consumers, family members, and mental health providers to oversee the mental health system. In fiscal year 2007, SAMHSA provided $401 million in block grants to states. According to a SAMHSA official, this made up an average of between 1 percent and 2 percent of each state's budget on community-based mental health services. SAMHSA also administers smaller targeted grants to support state mental health services and initiatives.

Part of SAMHSA's activities related to the block grant program are to promote specific practices—known as evidence-based practices—in mental health treatment. SAMHSA considers a practice evidence-based if it has been validated by research, such as clinical trials with experimental designs, and if it reflects expert opinion. On its Web site, SAMHSA provides toolkits for five types of evidence-based practices that states can use to design their programs. These five practices are Illness Management and Recovery, Assertive Community Treatment, Supported Employment, Family Psychoeducation, and Co-Occurring Disorders: Integrated Dual Disorders Treatment. (See app. III for details about these practices.)[14] SAMHSA is also promoting research on evidence-based practices in a number of other areas, including supported education, and plans on providing toolkits or other informational materials for these as well. A condition for receiving Community Mental Health Services Block Grant funds is that states are required by SAMHSA to report on whether they are using the evidence-based practices. In addition, states can use Medicaid funds to pay for certain services associated with the use of evidence-based practices.[15]

Education and Employment- Related Programs

Other federal programs fund educational and employment-related supports through states, localities, or other groups to individuals with a mental health disability. (See table 2.)

Through special education programs funded with federal dollars in part, students through age 21 with emotional disturbances and students with other disabilities with behavioral and emotional components can receive an individually tailored program of specialized instruction and support services set out in an individualized education program (IEP).[16] On the basis of decisions of the student's IEP team, students can receive such services as psychological services, counseling and social work services, and job coaching (as part of services supporting the transition of a student to post-school activities).

Another example of a program that provides educational and employment-related supports is Labor's WIA Youth Activities program, which funds efforts related to workforce training, education attainment, community involvement, and leadership development for low-income individuals aged 14 to 21 who have difficulty completing their education or securing or maintaining employment. Once they are determined to be WIA eligible, youth receive an assessment of their academic level, skills, and service needs. Local youth programs then use the assessment to create individualized service strategies, which lay out employment goals, educational objectives, and necessary services. In 2006, Labor received approximately $940 million in funding appropriated for WIA youth-related activities.

Table 2. Examples of Federal Programs That Can Provide Educational or Employment-Related Services to Young Adults with Serious Mental Illness

Department	Program	Purpose
Education	Rehabilitation Services—Vocational Rehabilitation Grants to States	Provide vocational rehabilitation services to persons with disabilities who are interested in seeking employment
	Individuals with Disabilities Education Act, Part B, Grants to States, Formula Grant Program	Provide special education and related services to children with disabilities to ensure they have available a free appropriate public education and to prepare them for further education, employment, and independent living
HHS	Chafee Foster Care Independence Program	Help current and former foster care youth achieve self-sufficiency through education, employment, financial management, housing, counseling, and other support
	Chafee Education and Training Vouchers Program	Provide vouchers to foster care youth adopted after age 16 or certain former foster care youth through funds of up to $5,000 per year for postsecondary education and training
Labor	Job Corps	Education and job training program for at-risk youth to prepare them for stable, long-term employment
	Workforce Investment Act (WIA) Youth Activities	Provide workforce training, educational activities, and leadership development opportunities to low-income youth
	YouthBuild	Provide disadvantaged youth with opportunities for employment, education, leadership development, and training through the construction and rehabilitation of permanent affordable housing for homeless individuals and low-income families

Source: GAO analysis.

Education's Rehabilitation Services Administration provides grants to assist state vocational rehabilitation agencies in providing employment- related services for individuals with disabilities, including individuals with serious mental illness. Vocational rehabilitation agencies assist individuals in pursuing gainful employment commensurate with their abilities and capabilities. Money for vocational rehabilitation is allotted to states and territories according to a formula, and over $2.8 billion was appropriated to states in 2007.

Finally, current and former foster care youth can receive services up to the age of 21 through the Chafee Foster Care Independence program. This program funds independent living, education, and training and gives states the flexibility to extend Medicaid coverage for former foster care youth up to age 21. Federal funding associated with these activities totaled $140 million in 2006.[17] However, we have found that there are critical gaps in mental health and housing services for foster youth and that states were serving less than half of their eligible foster care population through their programs.[18]

Programs that Provide Housing Supports

Other programs provide housing supports. (See table 3.) These programs range in scope, targeting low-income people generally to vulnerable groups specifically, such as the disabled or the homeless.

Table 3. Examples of Federal Programs That CanProvide Housing Support to Young Adults with Serious Mental Illness

Department	Program	Purpose
HHS	Runaway and Homeless Youth Grant Program	Provide street-based educational and prevention services and outreach to homeless and runaway youth who have been subjected to, or are at risk of being subjected to, sexual abuse, prostitution, or sexual exploitation
HUD	Public and Indian Housing	Provide and operate cost-effective, decent, safe, and affordable dwellings for lower -income families
	Section 8 Housing Choice Vouchers	Assist very low-income families to afford decent, safe, and sanitary rental housing

Table 3. (Continued).

Department	Program	Purpose
	Shelter Plus Care	Provide rental assistance to persons with disabilities (primarily those with serious mental illness, chronic problems with alcohol or drugs or both, acquired immunodeficiency syndrome, or related diseases) and their families in connection with supportive services funded from other sources
	Supportive Housing Programs	Develop supportive housing and services that will allow homeless persons to live as independently as possible
	Supportive Housing for Persons with Disabilities	Allow very low-income persons with disabilities to live as independently as possible in the community in affordable housing

Source: GAO analysis.

In: Young Adults with Serious Mental Illness ISBN: 978-1-60692-641-3
Editor: David O. Sullivan

Chapter 3

MORE THAN 2 MILLION YOUNG ADULTS HAVE A SERIOUS MENTAL ILLNESS THAT CAN AFFECT THEIR EDUCATION AND EMPLOYMENT

We estimate that at least 2.4 million young adults had a serious mental illness in 2006. This estimate is likely to be low because it is based on a survey that did not include individuals who were homeless, institutionalized, or incarcerated—populations that likely suffer high rates of mental illness. Most young adults with serious mental illness suffer from multiple disorders, and relative to young adults with no mental illness, they have significantly lower rates of high school graduation and postsecondary education. Our analysis also found that about 186,000 young adults received disability benefits from SSA in 2006 because their mental illness was so severe that they were found to be unable to engage in substantial gainful activity. Finally, although we were unable to identify the number of young adults with serious mental illness who were homeless or involved in the justice or foster care systems, research suggests that these groups have high rates of mental illness overall.

At Least 2.4 Million Young Adults Had a Serious Mental Illness in 2006, and Many Suffered from Multiple Disorders and Did Not Graduate from High School

According to our analysis of the NCS-R, an estimated 2.4 million young adults aged 18 through 26 had a serious mental illness in 2006— approximately 6.5 percent of the estimated 37 million young adults living in U.S. households.[19] We estimate that another 9.3 million—25.3 percent—had a moderate or mild mental illness, and that overall, nearly one in three young adults experienced some degree of mental illness in 2006. (See fig. 1.)

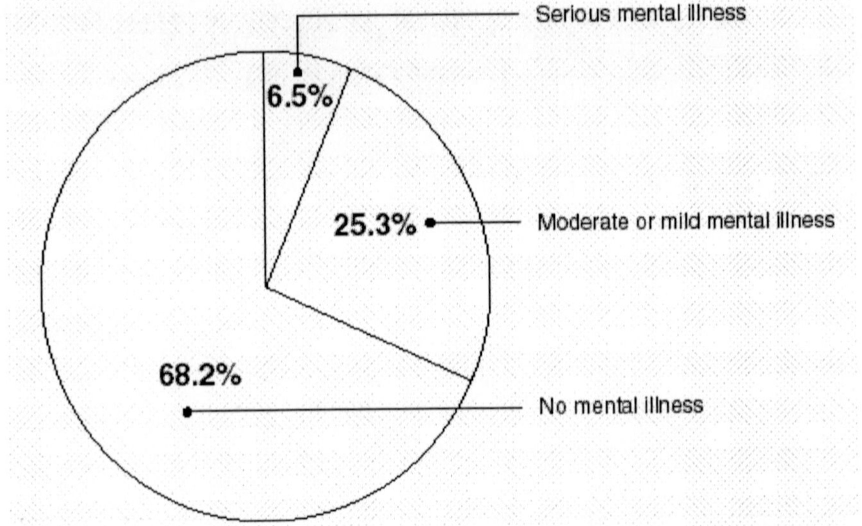

Source: GAO analysis of the National Comorbidity Survey Replication (NCS-R), 2001-2003.

Figure 1. Estimated Prevalence of Mental Illness among Young Adults Aged 18 through 26 in 2006, by Severity.

Because of limitations in the populations surveyed by the NCS-R, our estimated prevalence of serious mental illness among young adults in 2006 is likely to be low. Because only individuals living in households and campus housing were included in the sample population, individuals who were institutionalized, incarcerated, or homeless are not included in NCSR data.[20]

Research has shown that young adults in these populations may have significant rates of serious mental illness. The NCS-R may also under- represent the prevalence of serious mental illness because some individuals may not have reported what they believe will be viewed as socially unacceptable behaviors or may have chosen not to participate in the survey at all.[21] Finally, the NCS-R does not attempt to measure the prevalence of schizophrenia and other nonaffective psychotic disorders, and for this reason, may only represent a subset of those who would be considered by SAMHSA to meet the criteria for having a serious mental illness.[22]

Our analysis of the NCS-R indicates that certain disorders were most common among the young adult population aged 18 through 26 with serious mental illness. Specifically, we found that six mental disorders affected more than 25 percent of young adults with serious mental illness. The most prevalent of these was intermittent explosive disorder, and the other five were major depressive disorder, specific phobia, bipolar disorder, alcohol abuse, and social phobia.[23] (See table 4.) We also found that nearly all young adults with serious mental illness were diagnosed with more than one mental disorder. Specifically, 89 percent had two or more diagnoses and 56 percent had four or more.[24] For example, 20 percent of individuals with the most common diagnosis, intermittent explosive disorder, were also diagnosed with bipolar disorder, while 39 percent were also diagnosed with alcohol abuse. Results of the survey also suggest that about 32 percent of young adults with a serious mental illness had a co-occurring diagnosis of alcohol or drug abuse or dependence along with at least one other mental disorder.[25]

Table 4. Estimated Prevalence of Commonly Diagnosed Mental Illnesses among Young Adults Aged 18-26 with Serious Mental Illnesses

Disorder (past 12 months)	Characterization of disorder	Percent with disordera
Intermittent explosive disorder	Discrete episodes of a failure to resist aggressive impulses that result in serious violent acts or destruction of property	45
Major depressive disorder	Prolonged feelings of sadness, worthlessness, or irritability, often accompanied by behavioural changes, such as decreased energy or apathy	32
Specific phobia	Irrational fear associated with a specific object or situation	32

Table 4. (Continued).

Disorder (past 12 months)	Characterization of disorder	Percent with disordera
Bipolar disorderb	Mood swings ranging from high periods of mania to low periods of severe depression	28
Social phobia	Extreme anxiety in social situations	28
Alcohol abuse	Pattern of repeated alcohol use resulting in adverse consequences	26

Source: National Institutes of Health, DSM-IV, and GAO analysis of the NCS-R, 2001-2003

[a] All diagnoses were based on criteria specified in the DSM-IV for mental disorders occurring within the past 12 months, and all estimates are subject to a sampling error of within plus or minus 8 percentage points, with the exception of intermittent explosive disorder (plus or minus 13 percentage points), alcohol abuse and social phobia (plus or minusl 0 percentage points). The NCS-R measured rates of mental illness in U.S. households, and did not include individuals who are institutionalized, incarcerated, or homeless.

[b] The NCS-R provides separate prevalence estimates for bipolar I and bipolar II disorder. For the purposes of this analysis, we added the estimates together to derive the prevalence of bipolar disorder generally.

Young adults with serious mental illness had significantly lower rates of high school graduation than other young adults, according to our analysis of demographic information in the NCS-R. Specifically, the percentage of young adult respondents with serious mental illness who graduated high school was significantly lower than the percentage of those with moderate, mild, or no mental illnesses. Additionally, the percentage of young adult respondents with serious mental illness who continued their education after high school was also significantly lower than the percentage of those with moderate, mild, or no mental illness. (See figure 2.)

Young adults with serious mental illness also had lower rates of employment than other young adults, although the differences were not statistically significant, according to our analysis of the NCS-R. Specifically, 63 percent of young adults with serious mental illness reported they were currently employed, versus 68 percent of those with a mild or moderate mental illness and 71 percent of those with no mental illness.

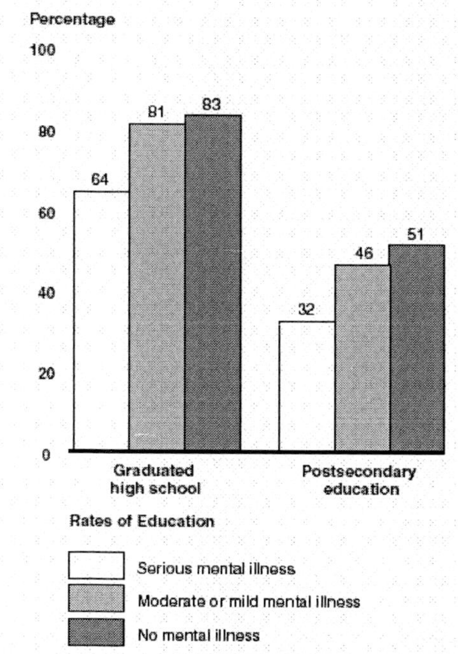

Source: GAO analysis of the National Comorbidity Survey Replication (NCS-R), 2001-2003

Note: Differences in estimates of education between young adults with serious mental illness and young adults with moderate, mild, or no mental illness are statistically significant at the 5 percent significance level and are subject to a sampling error of within plus or minus 12 percentage points. The NCS-R measured rates of mental illness in U.S. households and did not include individuals who are institutionalized, incarcerated, or homeless.

Figure 2. Rates of Education among Young Adults, Aged 18-26.

Results of other studies, however, suggest that unemployment is a common problem for young adults with serious mental illness. For example, an analysis of the 1994--95 National Health Interview Survey on Disability found an employment rate of 34 percent among working-age adults with mental health disabilities, versus 79 percent among adults with no disability.[26] In addition, the President's New Freedom Commission on Mental Health stated in its 2003 report that only one in three persons with a disability resulting from mental illness is employed.[27] (See app. IV for more detailed demographics of young adults with serious mental illness compared to those with moderate, mild, or no mental illness.)

About 186,000 Young Adults Had a Mental Illness So Severe that They Received Disability Benefits from the SSA in 2006

In 2006, about 186,000 young adults had a mental illness that was severe enough that they received disability payments from SSI, DI or both, meaning that they were found to be unable to engage in substantial, gainful activity because of their illness, according to our analysis of the TRF. The 186,000 individuals who received benefits in 2006 represented just under a quarter of all young adults who received SSI or DI that year and do not include individuals who receive benefits because of abnormalities in cognition or intellectual functioning, such as mental retardation or autism.[28] Of these young adults, about 67 percent received payments through SSI only, nearly 9 percent received payments from DI only, and 24 percent received concurrent payments from both programs. Among those receiving SSI payments, nearly 60 percent first became eligible before the age of 18.

The mental illnesses that were most common among young adults receiving payments from SSI, DI, or both for serious mental illness include schizophrenic, paranoid, and other functional psychotic disorders and affective mood disorders, such as depression or bipolar disorder. (See table 5.)

Table 5. Estimated Prevalence of Mental Disorders among Young Adults Aged 18- 26 Receiving SSI or DI or Both Because of a Serious Mental Illness

Disorder	Percent with disorder
Affective mood disorders	46
Schizophrenic, paranoid, and other functional psychotic disorders	33
Anxiety disorders	8
Personality disorders	5
Other mental disorders	8

Note: This analysis does not include those who receive disability benefits because of abnormalities in cognition or intellectual functioning, such as mental retardation or autism, or those whose eligibility has not been redetermined after turning 18.

Source: GAO analysis of SSA's Ticket Research File, 2006.

These young adults receiving SSI or DI or both scored lower on certain socioeconomic indicators than the general population of those with serious mental illness. Specifically, when we compared SSI and DI recipients with serious mental illness with their counterparts from the NCS-R, we found that the SSI and DI recipients had lower rates of high school graduation and employment. (See table 6.)

Table 6. Estimated Education, Employment, and Income for Young Adults Receiving SSI or DI Because of a Serious Mental Illness Compared to the General Population of Young Adults with Serious Mental Illness

Characteristic	SSI and DI recipients	All with a serious mental illness
Graduated high school	52%	64%
Currently employed	15%	63%
Average annual household income	$20,685	$45,667

Source: GAO analysis of SSA's National Beneficiary Survey, 2004, for estimates for SSI and DI recipients, and the National Comorbidity Survey Replication (NCS-R), 2001-2003, for estimates of all young adults with a serious mental illness.

Note: Our analysis of SSI and DI recipients does not include those who receive disability benefits because of abnormalities in cognition or intellectual functioning, such as mental retardation or autism. All estimates are subject to a sampling error of within plus or minus 12 percentage points for estimates from the NCS-R and plus or minus 7 percentage points for estimates from the NBS.

In addition, while 59 percent of those receiving disability payments reported having ever worked, only 15 percent reported being currently employed. This compares with an estimated 63 percent rate of employment for those in the NCS-R.[29] Finally, we found that SSI/DI recipients also had a lower average annual household income than all young adults with serious mental illness represented in the NCS-R. (See app. V for more detailed demographic analysis of young adults enrolled in SSI and DI due to serious mental illness.)

The number of young adults whose mental illness is severe enough to qualify for SSI or DI is likely to be higher than the 186,000 who were receiving disability payments in 2006 for two reasons. First, there could be some number of individuals who suffer from a serious mental illness who do not apply for SSI or DI or complete the application process. The process of proving eligibility requires the submission of medical records to document the medical nature of the mental illness, probable duration of the symptoms, and the degree of impairment the illness imposes, as well as proof of income for SSI eligibility—a process that might prove too difficult for those with a serious mental illness.[30] The second reason the 186,000 might not represent all who could qualify for disability benefits is that, according to SSA officials, some individuals who have a serious mental illness may be receiving benefits because of another disability, such as mental retardation, or a physical disability.[31] Our analysis of SSA administrative data found about 100,000 young adults whose primary disability was not a serious mental illness had a secondary diagnosis of a mental illness, which may have been severe enough, by itself, to qualify the individual for disability benefits. These individuals were therefore not included in our count of 186,000.

The Number of Young Adults with Serious Mental Illness Who Are Homeless or Involved in the Justice or Foster Care Systems is Unknown, Although Research Suggests Their Rates of Mental Illness May Be High

We were not able to estimate the number of young adults in certain vulnerable populations who have a serious mental illness, although the available research suggests that rates of mental illness are high in these groups. These vulnerable populations include young adults transitioning out of the foster care system—who may have limited family support for their struggle with serious mental illness—and young adults who become homeless or incarcerated. The NCS-R does not include individuals who are homeless or incarcerated, and although individuals in foster care are included, they are not specifically identified as such in the data. Additionally, a review of literature on homelessness and the justice and foster care systems yielded no studies that produced national estimates of the number of such young adults in those groups. Studies that examine mental illness in those groups either do not yield estimates specific to young adults or do not measure serious mental illness in a consistent way that can be compared across groups.

Although the prevalence of serious mental illness has not been studied in these young adult populations nationally, available research suggests that their rates of mental illness may be high. With respect to young adults in foster care, a national survey that included 464 individuals aged 12 to 17 who had been placed in foster care found that they were about four times more likely to have attempted suicide in the preceding year when compared to those never placed in foster care. In addition, they were about three times more likely to have experienced significant anxiety and mood symptoms, such as depression or mania.[32] Research also indicates that mental health problems among foster care children may persist into adulthood. For example, the Northwest Foster Care Alumni Study, which assessed 659 adults aged 20 through 33 in Oregon and Washington who had been in foster care as children, found that over half had experienced symptoms of one or more mental disorders in the previous year, and 20 percent had symptoms of three or more mental disorders.[33] The study compared these results to results from the NCS-R for adults in the same age range, which found that only three percent of adults in that age range had symptoms of 3 or more disorders in the previous year.

Studies also suggest high rates of mental illness among young adults who are homeless. For example, an Urban Institute study based on the National Survey of Homeless Assistance Providers and Clients estimated that 46 percent of homeless individuals aged 20 through 24 had experienced a mental health problem in the prior year.[34] Another study of 432 homeless young people in Los Angeles found that 63 percent of those aged 19 through 24 currently had depressive symptoms and 38 percent had attempted suicide at some point in their lives.[35]

Finally, studies have found that young adults involved in the criminal justice system have high rates of mental illness. According to two national surveys conducted by the Bureau of Justice Statistics, 62.6 percent of young adults aged 24 or younger in state prisons had a mental health problem in 2004, and 70.3 percent of those in local jails had a mental health problem in 2002.[36] Further, a multi-state survey funded by DOJ's Office of Juvenile Justice and Delinquency Prevention found that about 70 percent of youth involved with the juvenile justice system had at least one mental health disorder, and 27 percent had a severe mental health disorder in 2006.[37]

In: Young Adults with Serious Mental Illness ISBN: 978-1-60692-641-3
Editor: David O. Sullivan

Chapter 4

Young Adults with Serious Mental Illness Face Challenges Accessing Appropriate Support

According to researchers, public officials, and advocates, young adults with serious mental illness can have difficulty finding services tailored to their needs, qualifying for adult programs, and navigating multiple programs and delivery systems. While these young adults need a range of support services, the existing public mental health, employment, and housing programs are not necessarily tailored to their disability or their stage of life, which may lead them to forgo services entirely. Further, young adults who received free or low-cost mental health services as children generally face different, and sometimes more stringent, eligibility requirements as adults. Finally, federal officials and researchers have recognized the difficulties this group and their families have in navigating the broad array of programs that can help meet their needs.

Public Services Are Often Not Tailored to the Needs of Young Adults with Serious Mental Illness

Although appropriate mental health services are a key to achieving independence, researchers and officials told us that these services are often not tailored to the age-related needs of the young adult population. We have previously reported that directors of programs serving youth aged 14 through 24 have difficulty finding adequate age-appropriate mental health services for their clients.[38] A national expert has noted that adult mental health service providers in one state, for example, were generally not trained in adolescent development and so were unprepared to treat young adults with serious mental illness who tend to be relatively psychosocially immature.[39] Officials in three of the states we visited similarly reported a need for better training among mental health providers in issues related to young adults. Other researchers have noted that group therapy should involve members in the same age range, given that young adults' self-esteem can depend significantly on peer acceptance. However, young adults are often referred to group-oriented treatment that may include mainly older adults who do not share their transition-age issues and is therefore often inappropriate for them, according to mental health advocates with whom we spoke.[40]

While young adults with serious mental illness can benefit from a variety of employment programs, these programs are also not necessarily tailored to the particular needs of this population. For example, state officials in three of the four states we visited told us that WIA Youth centers in those states often lack the expertise to help young adults with serious mental illness find appropriate employment because these centers generally do not have the capacity to provide the intensive and customized support these individuals need. Labor officials told us that, as a result, WIA staff often refer youth they believe have mental illness to vocational rehabilitation programs. However, according to federal officials, vocational rehabilitation programs have been traditionally used by those with physical disabilities and are also not always designed to meet mental health needs.[41] Advocates working with young adults in most states we visited likewise noted that the vocational rehabilitation services available to the youth they work with have not been responsive to their mental health-related issues. Similarly, officials in one state noted that service providers for students with disabilities at colleges and universities often lack the expertise and training to support students with serious mental illness.[42]

Finally, while researchers noted that young adults with serious mental illnesses experience difficulty living independently and in some cases finding housing, officials in all of the states we visited cited the inability to find appropriate housing as a key problem for this population. Specifically, they noted that there are not enough permanent housing options that are targeted to this age group. Supportive housing--which often includes a comprehensive set of supports such as job training and mental health services--is recommended by SAMHSA as a resource for those with mental illness. However, officials in all states we visited said there was a lack of such housing available. Additionally, where supportive housing is available, it is not necessarily geared to young adults. For example,

HUD officials reported that the median age of the head of households receiving HUD supportive housing is 47. One service provider explained that if housing options are not geared to their age group, young adults with serious mental illness may end up homeless.

Researchers and advocates have noted that if services are not suited to their age or disability, young adults with serious mental illness may choose not to participate. Young adults are particularly sensitive to the stigma associated with receiving treatment for their symptoms, and SAMHSA has reported that they have the lowest "help-seeking behavior" of any age group.[43] Furthermore, as they age into the adult mental health system, their parents are generally no longer responsible for their mental health treatment, and these young adults then have the option to decline treatment. In Massachusetts, for example, a state official found that, in one locality, more than half of the young adults who had received mental health services as children chose not to receive them as adults. She attributed this to a lack of services geared to their disability and age.

DIFFERENCES IN ELIGIBILITY CRITERIA BETWEEN CHILD AND ADULT SYSTEMS POSE CHALLENGES

Researchers and state officials we spoke with noted that young adults who once received public mental health services, Medicaid, or SSI or DI as children face different and sometimes more restrictive eligibility requirements for these programs as adults. They added that ineligibility for these adult programs can end established relationships with mental health professionals or otherwise disrupt receipt of mental health services.

Qualifying for free or low-cost mental health services is often more difficult for adults than children. The National Conference of State Legislatures found that, among state programs, the clinical criteria for receiving adult public mental health services are generally narrower for adults than for children.[44] Another study has found that in 2001 adult and child mental health policies were different in 34 states, and in 31 of those states, the range of qualifying disorders was more limited for adults than for children.[45] Specifically, in half of the states with different criteria, the adult requirement was more restrictive by virtue of citing fewer specific diagnoses to qualify. Similarly, in most states children can qualify for Medicaid---the major federal funder of public mental health services---at higher household income levels than adults, who must also meet other categorical eligibility criteria. In these states, a young person previously covered by Medicaid as a child who becomes an adult risks losing access to the mental health treatment and psychiatric rehabilitation services covered by the program. Advocates, state officials, and researchers all cited the loss of Medicaid benefits because of different eligibility requirements between children and adults as a challenge for young adults with serious mental illness.

When youth receiving SSI are evaluated using adult rules for SSI within one year of turning age 18, as required by law, they also find that the adult eligibility criteria are different and can result in a cessation of payments. This can also lead to a loss of Medicaid eligibility. SSA officials told us that 25 percent of youth who received SSI because of a mental health--related condition do not qualify for SSI once they turn 18. Advocates working with these young adults and their families in the states we visited cited this loss of SSI benefits as a key concern for young adults with serious mental illness in their transition to adulthood. SSA officials indicated that the loss of benefits for these young adults resulted partly from the fact that certain mental disorders that are considered disabling to children are not applicable to adults.[46] For example, adult disorders that qualify for SSI do not include eating disorders and attention deficit hyperactivity disorder. However, SSA officials told us that they are currently working on revising some of the criteria for mental health impairments so that the criteria for children and adults are more closely aligned.

Navigating Multiple Programs and Systems Can also Present Challenges

Because young adults with serious mental illness usually have a number of needs requiring multiple supports, they can find it difficult to receive all the services they need when programs are administered by different agencies with varying eligibility requirements. Given their multiple needs, a coordinated set of benefits is important for a successful transition to adulthood. Labor recently reported, however, that there is no single system that guides youth, in general, through the process of becoming productive, self-sufficient adults and that existing services for them are uncoordinated.[47] Bazelon has similarly found that the programs serving young adults with mental illness have varying age and income requirements and may use different definitions of mental illness, which can make it difficult to obtain multiple services.[48] In addition, according to state officials with whom we visited, program staff may not collaborate with or notify one another of the service plans they develop for clients. For example, the director of a mental health advocacy organization in Massachusetts told us that when a young person has a serious mental illness and the secondary school is involved, the staff at the school will typically not speak with the young person's doctor or Medicaid provider in order to coordinate behavior plans or more fully understand the particular mental illness.

Navigating the varying eligibility requirements and service plans of multiple programs across a number of delivery systems can be difficult for anyone, but young adults with serious mental illness may have fewer interpersonal and emotional resources with which to do so. Mental health advocates told us that because young adults with serious mental illness tend to be involved in different service delivery systems, their parents or other caring adults must often operate as their de facto case worker, attempting to organize and coordinate various services. However, researchers and family advocates have also found that a major challenge for these parents and caring adults is their need for information related to availability of supports. For example, one researcher found that families wanted information related to the young adults' condition and treatment, available community resources, and supports for caregivers and that they generally reported feeling overwhelmed by the complexity of the system of agencies and organizations.

In: Young Adults with Serious Mental Illness ISBN: 978-1-60692-641-3
Editor: David O. Sullivan

Chapter 5

SELECTED STATES PROVIDE MULTIDIMENSIONAL SERVICES TO YOUNG ADULTS WITH SERIOUS MENTAL ILLNESS USING VARIOUS STRATEGIES

Recognizing the challenges faced by young adults with serious mental illness, the four states we visited—Connecticut, Maryland, Massachusetts, and Mississippi—have designed programs with multidimensional services to help them transition into adulthood. States have used various strategies to provide these services. They include broadening eligibility criteria for mental health services, employing some of the evidence-based practices promoted by SAMHSA, coordinating efforts across multiple state agencies, leveraging federal and state funding sources, and involving consumers and family members in developing policies and aligning services.

STATES WE VISITED HAVE PROGRAMS PROVIDING MULTIDIMENSIONAL SERVICES TO YOUNG ADULTS

The four states we selected for review have developed programs that provide multidimensional services to young adults with serious mental illness.[49] Administered by their respective mental health agencies, these programs are implemented at the local level generally by mental health authorities, non-profit organizations, and community-based mental health providers. In addition to health care services, the programs provide a range of services intended to be age and developmentally appropriate, including vocational rehabilitation, employment, life-skills development, and, in some cases, housing. These four states try to tailor these services so that, to the extent possible, young adults receive services appropriate for each individual's transition needs.[50] They also try to integrate the services so that young adults do not have to navigate multiple discrete programs. Tailoring and integrating services are both central tenets of the wraparound approach. In Connecticut, the young adult program initially focused on individuals referred from the Department of Children and Families, but has since evolved to focus on a broader group of young adults with serious mental illness.[51] This focus is similar to that of the other states' programs.

The young adult programs administered by these four states vary in the number of young adults with serious mental illness that they serve and have not yet been systematically evaluated for their effectiveness. For example, in state fiscal year 2007, Connecticut's specialized program for young adults with serious mental illness aged 18 through 25 served 716 individuals, or about 27 percent of the 2,615 young adults with serious mental illness receiving mental health services from the state mental health agency. State officials explained that not every young adult needs the kinds of intensive services provided under the state's specialized program for young adults but added that many more young adults could benefit from the program than are currently being served.

In 2007, Massachusetts's young adult program served all of the approximately 2,600 young adults aged 16 to 25 with serious mental illness in the state's mental health system, providing one or more services, including case management, housing, employment, education, and peer mentoring. A smaller number received a variety of other mental health and social services. Although most of the states' young adult programs have existed for more than five years, none of the states have systematically collected data on outcomes to evaluate the effectiveness of their programs. State officials said that their budget resources are limited and they have focused on providing services. (See app. VII for a description of the four state programs.)

States We Visited Use a Number of Strategies to Provide Services

In the four states we visited, state officials described a variety of strategies they have used to provide multidimensional services to young adults with serious mental illness. The strategies include broadening eligibility criteria for mental health services, employing evidence-based practices promoted by SAMHSA, coordinating efforts across multiple state agencies, leveraging federal and state funding sources, and involving consumers and family members in developing policies and aligning services.

Broadening Eligibility Criteria for Mental Health Services

Maryland has chosen to broaden eligibility criteria for mental health services for young adults beyond the medical necessity criteria established for adults with serious mental illness. Specifically, Maryland generally limits its comprehensive adult mental health services to individuals with certain diagnoses and functional limitations, but state officials have approved eligibility for young adults who do not meet all the criteria. Maryland officials told us they aim to identify and treat individuals so that they can become meaningful community participants rather than becoming dependent on the service system. They said that state services target young adults who are in or at risk of out-of-home placement, such as in residential treatment centers. Many of these young adults have histories of severe trauma, have limited community living skills, and have increased psychotic symptoms.

Employing Evidenced-Based Practices

Another strategy is to deliver multidimensional services using evidence-based practices promoted by SAMHSA. Although these evidence-based practices have not been empirically tested specifically on the young adult population, states we visited are using some of them. Some of these practices involve bringing integrated mental health and social services to the young adults living in the community rather than expecting them to navigate multiple discrete programs on their own. For example, Massachusetts and Connecticut have used the Assertive Community Treatment model, which employs an interdisciplinary team of psychiatrists, social workers, and nurses to provide psychiatric, rehabilitation, and other support services in the community 24 hours per day.[52] In this model, team members collaborate to tailor services on an individual basis, taking into account cultural diversity.[53] Assertive Community Treatment services are designed for individuals who have the most serious symptoms of mental illness and greatest impairment in functioning. They often come to the program in crisis or upon release from inpatient psychiatric care. In Massachusetts, the Assertive

Community Treatment services are available in various locations throughout the state, including in three sites in the Southeastern Area that specifically target these services for young adults. Connecticut uses this treatment model in some of its young adult program sites, often to serve those leaving foster care and the juvenile justice system.

Connecticut, Maryland, and Massachusetts provide another evidence- based practice—supported employment—to assist young adults with serious mental illness. Based on the principle that work is therapeutic, supported employment programs are designed to help individuals work in competitive jobs in the community while receiving mental health treatment and rehabilitation services. These programs focus on rapid job placement in competitive employment. Once the individual is working, the program provides supports to retain employment. In Maryland, for example, the state mental health agency and the state vocational rehabilitation agency approved 30 evidenced-based supported employment programs available for young adults with serious mental illness, although these are not uniformly distributed across the state.[54] According to state officials, these programs help individuals find and maintain meaningful jobs that are consistent with the individual's preferences and abilities.

In addition, Connecticut has been providing a type of support that SAMHSA is beginning to explore as a potential evidence-based practice— supported education for young adults with serious mental illness who enroll in higher education. The Connecticut mental health agency provides funding for a supported education counselor at one of the state universities, who provides case management services, acts as a liaison between the university's disability office and the student with mental illness, and helps students work with relevant university staff to get appropriate accommodations for their mental illness in the classroom or during exams. This counselor serves also as an information resource for the student's parents, university faculty, and personnel that work with the young adult, as well as local mental health authorities and other key persons in the mental health system across the state.[55]

Coordinating Services Across State Agencies

Agencies in states we visited are also coordinating to develop policy and provide multidimensional services. Agencies coordinate client referral, eligibility determination, and service delivery. These coordination efforts help address eligibility gaps between the children and adult mental health systems and ease service delivery so that young adults do not have to navigate multiple discrete programs.

- *Formal Referral Process across Agencies*: This strategy can provide a bridge for individuals who were receiving services and supports from one agency as children but must transition to another agency in order to continue to receive those services and supports as adults. In Connecticut, many young adults are formally referred to the Connecticut mental health agency by the state agency responsible for foster care, juvenile justice, and youth mental health services. A cooperative agreement between the two agencies specifies appropriate candidates for the state mental health agency's young adult program, the process for providing services to them by both agencies during the transition period, and the agencies' respective funding responsibilities. Transitioning youth are referred as early as possible, generally at age 16, to allow state mental health agency officials to develop appropriate plans. These referrals are made on a monthly basis.
- *Integrated Eligibility Determination and Service Delivery*: Maryland's mental health agency has a formal arrangement with the state's vocational rehabilitation agency to integrate eligibility determination and service delivery processes. Under a cooperative agreement signed by the two agencies in 2007, individuals determined eligible by the mental health agency are also determined eligible by the vocational rehabilitation agency for supported employment services. The two agencies have automated their eligibility determination processes to be simultaneous. Once approved for services, individuals receive assistance finding and keeping a job and managing their mental illness in the workplace. Services are provided by not-for-profit supported employment programs that hire employment support specialists, according to a state mental health official.
- *Use of Statewide and Local Interagency Task Forces*: In 2003, Mississippi's mental health agency created an interagency Transitional Services Task Force to develop policies and identify resources appropriate for young adults with serious mental illness aged 14 through 25.[56] The task force monitors the implementation of the state's young adult program at its two current sites and hopes to eventually present the results of an evaluation to justify expansion of the program statewide. At the local level, Mississippi established Multidisciplinary Assessment and Planning Teams, comprised of local officials from various state agencies

and advocates that meet and review cases that include individuals aged 14 to 21 transitioning from the child to adult mental health systems, as well as other young adults considered high-risk. Currently operating in 33 of 82 counties in the state, the teams coordinate delivery of various services including mental health, education, vocational rehabilitation, and health care services.[57] They have some flexible funds for providing additional multidimensional services, such as housing, tutoring, school uniforms, and in-home respite care.

Leveraging Federal and State Funding Resources

Another strategy is to leverage federal and state funds to finance programs for young adults with serious mental illness. The four states we visited use Medicaid to pay for mental health services approved by CMS in the states' Medicaid plans, such as those provided in a physician's office, at an outpatient clinic, or rehabilitation program in the community. To varying extents, three of the four states—Maryland, Massachusetts, and Mississippi—use Medicaid's rehabilitation option to pay for additional services[58] that can support a young adult's recovery from mental illness. These services, which are provided to address daily problems related to community living and interpersonal relationships, may include psychiatric rehabilitation program services, symptom management, and counseling.[59] Further, some of these states have used certain CMS grants to help cover some expenses of their young adult programs. For example, Mississippi targeted the Real Choice Systems Change grant that it received from CMS in 2001 to develop a "person-centered planning" approach for delivering services to young adults with serious mental illness.[60] The grant concluded in 2004, but the state is using its own funds to provide these services in two of its local mental health centers and to provide training related to this approach. In addition, all four states we visited use their own funds to pay for mental health and other services for individuals in their young adult programs that are not eligible for Medicaid or who are Medicaid-eligible but receive services not covered under Medicaid.[61] Examples of such services include housing and transportation costs.

In addition, states we reviewed used funds from other federal programs to provide various transition services to eligible youth through their young adult programs. In the case of Maryland, this involves "braided funding" for supported employment services. Braided funding refers to the integration of funding streams from multiple agencies so that the individual receiving services experience a seamless array of services. For example, various components of supported employment services are funded by Maryland's mental health agency, Maryland's vocational rehabilitation, and Medicaid. Maryland's mental health agency and Maryland's vocational rehabilitation agency have a cooperative agreement that outlines the funding components. In addition, Maryland requires individuals in its public mental health system, including young adults, to apply for SSI or any other applicable public benefit in order to receive income assistance (to pay for housing and insurance) to pay for services, according to a state mental health official. In the development of its young adult program, Maryland also uses part of its CMS Medicaid Infrastructure Grant to consult with experts on funding strategies and to implement the web-based mental health and vocational rehabilitation eligibility system.

In addition to federal funds leveraged at the state level, some local state agencies obtain services for their clients from other federally funded programs. Officials from one service provider in Massachusetts told us that their organization works with state housing authorities to secure HUD's Section 8 Rental Voucher Program for adults who were previously homeless.[62] When we conducted our site visit, the provider was using 10 such vouchers to serve 20 to 30 young adults, according to this provider.[63] State officials said that this was an important initiative by this provider because states find it particularly difficult to obtain appropriate housing for young adults with serious mental illness who have criminal records. In Maryland, although the state mental health agency does not work directly with the state WIA Office, a local provider in its young adult program works with local WIA offices in two counties to coordinate employment services for young adults with serious mental illness. This provider stations case managers at these counties' WIA One-Stop Centers to help young adults with serious mental illness with tasks such as identifying job opportunities or scheduling interviews.[64]

Involving Young Adults and Their Families

Another strategy is to involve young adults and family members in developing policy and delivering and evaluating services. The Massachusetts mental health agency established a statewide Youth Development Committee in 2002 to focus on individuals aged 16 through 25 with serious mental illness. Committee membership includes young adults, parents, state child and adult mental health agency representatives, transition experts, and other professionals. Co-chaired by young adults with serious mental illness, the committee has engaged in a strategic planning process and meets every month to discuss progress in the field. The Committee has young adult representatives from all areas of the state, and these representatives report on progress related to supported employment, housing, and transition age youth case management in their areas. They also discuss Massachusetts's implementation of the Transition to Independence Process (TIP) system and identify emerging staff training needs associated with Motivational Interviewing and the TIP model. TIP is an approach that delivers individualized-tailored services to youth and young adults with serious mental illness by involving them in defining and achieving their employment, education, and community-life goals.[65] The state also has a Youth Leadership Academy, which young adults attend to build peer networks and social connections and obtain information on key topics such as substance abuse prevention and health insurance.

In: Young Adults with Serious Mental Illness
Editor: David O. Sullivan
ISBN: 978-1-60692-641-3

Chapter 6

Federal Agencies Have Supported Demonstrations, Provided Technical Assistance and Research, and Formed Interagency Working Groups

The needs of young adults with serious mental illness have also received some attention from the federal government, which has, to some extent, supported state efforts to serve them through demonstrations, technical assistance, and research. In response to presidential concern about uncoordinated service delivery in the mental health and other related systems, several federal agencies have formed working groups to consider opportunities for collaboration among programs that involve mental health, youth in transition, or the needs of transitional youth with disabilities.[66]

One Former Federal Demonstration Project Developed Transition Programs that Continue in Five States and States Can Use Other Federal Programs to Provide or Coordinate Services

SAMHSA, in collaboration with Education, funded local services through the Partnerships for Youth in Transition demonstration aimed at developing local programs and assisting young adults with serious mental illness as they transition to adulthood.[67] A total of $9.4 million was awarded over 4 years to several sites in Maine, Minnesota, Pennsylvania, Utah, and Washington. The demonstrations were intended to be self- sustaining and, although funding ended in 2006, sites in Pennsylvania, Utah and Washington have continued the program in total and aspects of the program continue in Minnesota and Maine. Pennsylvania, for example, has continued to operate a program serving young adults aged 14 through 25 in two economically disadvantaged communities. In these communities, young adults with serious mental illness continue to be involved in planning and implementing activities and serve on review panels and state- level advisory boards. These communities also use transition facilitators who work with young adults to help determine their goals and how local services can assist them.

SAMHSA officials stated that this demonstration project resulted in positive outcomes that they would like other states to achieve. A preliminary evaluation of 193 program participants conducted by the National Center on Youth in Transition at the University of South Florida suggests that there may be some positive outcomes, such as employment, for participants from the program after 1 year.[68] While the Partnerships for Youth in Transition demonstration ended in 2006, SAMHSA officials indicated they are considering continuing similar work and looking for opportunities to use the data and lessons learned from this demonstration to help states better serve young adults with serious mental illness.

While we found that there are currently no federal programs that target this population, agencies fund other demonstration projects that support state and local efforts to provide or better coordinate existing services for transition-age individuals. For example, SSA's Youth Transition Demonstration funds programs at ten sites that help youth aged 14 through 25, who receive or may qualify for SSI, transition from school to employment. SSA officials stated that mental illness is the primary disabling condition of 23 percent of the Youth Transition Demonstration enrollees. SSA developed alternative SSI rules only for the participants in this program that included extending their eligibility for SSI beyond age 18, even if the recipient does not meet SSI adult eligibility criteria. While not targeted to young adults with serious mental illness, CMS also offers a number of Medicaid demonstration waivers or options that can help states pay for services for this population. For example, the Community

Alternatives to Psychiatric Residential Treatment Facilities Demonstration Grant Program has awarded 5-year grants to 10 states aimed at preventing youth up to age 21 from entering psychiatric residential treatment facilities. This demonstration can cover the cost of a comprehensive package of community-based services for these youth, such as 24-hour support and crisis intervention, respite care for families, and after-school support programs. Additional federal programs that can be used by states to serve young adults with serious mental illness are described earlier in this report, as well as included in appendix VI.

Federal Agencies Provide Technical Assistance and Fund Research

Currently, some federal agencies provide technical assistance on promising practices that can help states coordinate services for young adults with serious mental illness as they transition to adulthood.

- SAMHSA's Center for Mental Health Services contracts with two nonprofit organizations to operate the *Technical Assistance Partnership for Child and Family Mental Health.* The Partnership facilitates collaboration among government officials, organizations, and community leaders to develop and implement systems of care. SAMHSA officials told us the Partnership has recently begun to provide information on the specific needs and issues pertinent to young adults with serious mental illness and resources on child welfare youth in transition.
- The *National Collaborative on Workforce and Disability for Youth,* funded by Labor's Office of Disability Employment Policy, provides technical assistance to One-Stop Centers to increase their capacity to serve youth aged 14 through 25 with disabilities, including those with serious mental illness. For example, according to Labor officials, Florida used this resource to enable its workforce development system to better assist youth with disabilities as they transition to adulthood. Recognizing the uncoordinated service delivery systems that youth must navigate, the Collaborative also published a resource guide for workforce practitioners and policy makers. The guide is designed to promote an understanding of how to serve youth with mental health needs and provides information on overcoming obstacles to better coordinate services across delivery systems for young adults with serious mental illness.[69]

With regard to federal support for research in this area, NIMH awarded a $1.1 million grant in 2007 to four research projects examining innovative strategies to provide services to youth with serious mental illness. According to NIMH, while evidence-based and traditional treatment models have been developed and tested for use with younger children and adults, evidence-based interventions and services have not been empirically tested on young adults or systematically adapted for this specific age group. The goal of three of the research projects is to assess the impact of tailoring existing treatment models to the needs of transition-aged youth. For example, one researcher is planning to adapt an established family-focused intervention approach for juvenile offenders to one that gives youth offenders with serious mental illness more control of their treatment and targets age-relevant social, work, and independent living skills. Another project examines young adults' use of primary care, mental health services, and psychotropic medications, as well as their overall mental health care costs. Agency officials told us information could help inform future research and strategies that promote continuity of care for young adults with serious mental illness as they transition to adulthood.[70]

FEDERAL INTERAGENCY GROUPS ARE BEGINNING TO COORDINATE MENTAL HEALTH SERVICES AND SERVICES FOR YOUTH IN TRANSITION AND YOUTH WITH DISABILITIES

Although there are no federal interagency coordination efforts that focus exclusively on young adults with serious mental illness, three independent multiagency groups were recently formed to consider opportunities to coordinate federal programs and could address the needs of this group. According to agency officials, while efforts are not coordinated across these three groups formally, they have similar agency and staff participation. Figure 3 lists these groups, their target population, goals, and participating agencies.

While interagency groups have been tasked with coordinating across agencies, officials from a number of agencies noted that differences in their missions and goals may make it difficult to coordinate services for young adults with serious mental illness. For example, according to one SAMHSA official, mental health agencies are more focused on maintaining youth in the home or in a community-based setting, whereas juvenile justice agencies are more focused on protecting the community from youth offenders. Agency officials also cited differences in eligibility criteria across programs as a challenge for coordination, stating that age requirements for receiving benefits—often written in statute—vary across some programs. Despite these limitations, ongoing federal coordination efforts are beginning to address the needs of this population.

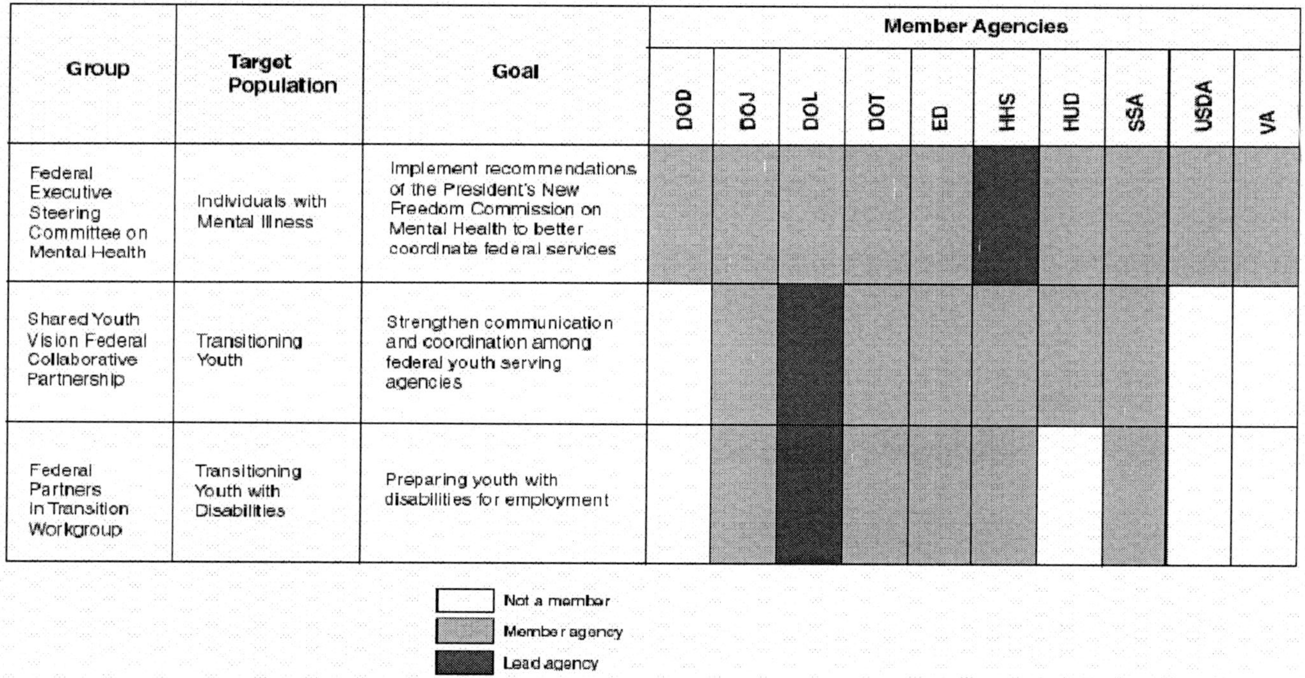

Source: GAO analysis.

Note: National Council on Disability and U.S. Equal Employment Opportunity Commission also participate in the Federal Partners in Transition Workgroup. Corporation for National and Community Service also participates in Shared Youth Vision Federal Collaborative Partnership. DOD = Department of Defense; DOT = Department of Transportation; VA = Veterans Administration.

Figure 3. Federal Coordination Efforts on Mental Health, Youth in Transition, and Transitioning Youth with Disabilities.

The Federal Executive Steering Committee on Mental Health was formed in response to the 2003 President's New Freedom Commission on Mental Health, which made recommendations to the federal government to better coordinate services, such as employment supports and housing, for those with mental illness. The committee has taken steps to promote access to supported employment services for young adults with serious mental illness by reviewing existing federal programs and initiatives for youth transitioning to the workforce to better coordinate their efforts. To promote youth leadership and youth-guided policymaking related to mental health at the federal level, the committee, led by Labor's Office of Disability Employment Policy, also held a National Youth Summit in 2007. The President's New Freedom Commission recommended actions to address mental health stigma, and SAMHSA launched a campaign specifically targeted to young adults.[71]

The Shared Youth Vision Federal Collaborative Partnership was created to strengthen coordination among federal youth-serving agencies. It was formed in response to a report written by the White House Task Force on Disadvantaged Youth in 2003, which identified challenges related to coordination among youth-serving programs and prompted federal efforts to support capacity building and collaboration among those agencies. Many of the federal officials we spoke with indicated this initiative could have an impact on young adults, including those with serious mental illness. Sixteen states have received funding through this initiative to develop interagency collaboration as well as state and local partnerships to provide transition assistance to disadvantaged young adults, including those with serious mental illness. For example, the Oklahoma Youth Vision Project is working across eight state youth-serving agencies, Job Corps, as well as local school districts, group homes, and employers to help disadvantaged youth, particularly those aging out of foster care, aged 16 through 21, graduate from high school and become employed.[72] In addition, this initiative sponsors technical assistance forums for participating federal agencies and runs a solutions desk that provides the 16 state grantees with a single point of access to federal resources such as training and technical assistance in implementing federal grants related to disadvantaged youth.

The third coordination initiative, Federal Partners in Transition Workgroup, led by Labor's Office of Disability Employment Policy, began in June 2005 and focuses exclusively on disabled youth transitioning to adulthood, including young adults with serious mental illness. The Federal Partners in Transition Workgroup brings together federal agency staff who work on youth, transition, and disability issues. This group has concentrated on strengthening connections with employers and preparing youth with disabilities for the labor market. It also plans to hold a forum in 2008 to coordinate federally funded transition-focused technical assistance centers across agencies.

Although none of these federal interagency coordination groups or existing programs focuses exclusively on young adults with serious mental illness, overall they are beginning to explore ways to coordinate and provide services to assist this group.

In: Young Adults with Serious Mental Illness ISBN: 978-1-60692-641-3
Editor: David O. Sullivan

Chapter 7

CONCLUDING OBSERVATIONS

State investments in programs to help young adults with serious mental illness become productive and independent are designed to address the challenges these individuals face. The state and local officials we spoke with appeared to be optimistic about the potential of efforts like theirs to make a difference for these young adults. The federal government has played a limited but important role in these efforts by funding demonstrations and research and providing technical assistance. Evaluations of these demonstration projects have shown some promising outcomes, and the number of practices grounded in evidence-based research continues to grow. While programs that assist transitional youth, youth with disabilities, and the mentally ill are situated in different departments, federal agencies are beginning to work together to coordinate these programs to better serve young adults with serious mental illness. The federal government's continuing efforts to disseminate information about promising state and local programs may sustain the momentum in this area by providing valuable lessons and encouragement to others interested in assisting young adults with serious mental illness.

In: Young Adults with Serious Mental Illness ISBN: 978-1-60692-641-3
Editor: David O. Sullivan

Chapter 8

RESPONSE TO AGENCY COMMENTS

We provided a draft of this report to Education, DOJ, HHS, HUD, Labor, and SSA and draft sections concerning their states to agencies in Connecticut, Maryland, Massachusetts, and Mississippi. We received technical comments from all of the federal and state agencies, which we incorporated where appropriate, and general comments from HHS, which are included in appendix XIII. In its general comments, HHS indicated that the report was pertinent and timely. However, HHS stated that the report should have included a number of other important topics and should have focused on younger individuals as well as those aged 18 through 26. While we agree that additional research could be beneficial, our report focused specifically on the objectives and population we agreed upon with our requesters. To better convey our scope, we revised the report title in response to HHS's suggestion.

HHS also commented that our definition of serious mental illness was unclear. In particular, they took issue with our use of the NCS-R to estimate the number of young adults with serious mental illness. They believe that data from the NCS-R represent only a subset of those individuals who would be considered to have a serious mental illness under the definition used by SAMHSA to determine how states can use Community Mental Health Block grant (see 58 *Fed. Reg.* 29422 (May 20, 1993), implementing Pub. L. 102-32 1). Specifically, they pointed out that the NCS-R does not include those in institutions and does not identify those with schizophrenia, or personality disorder. Additionally, HHS stated that the researchers and consumer organizations that we interviewed were weighted toward those with expertise in childhood mental illnesses and did not include experts in schizophrenia or adult mental health consumer organizations. HHS also stated that the report should have included a more extensive discussion of serious emotional disturbance and the degree to which states were providing services specifically for young adults with serious mental illness.

Researchers and policy makers have long recognized that defining serious mental illness in order to estimate its prevalence or to determine eligibility for services presents a significant challenge. Our report generally uses a definition of serious mental illness that is based on SAMHSA's regulation implementing Pub. L. 102-321. We clarified the text to explain that in places throughout the report, we may use a slightly broader or narrower concept of serious mental illness as necessitated by available data as well as programmatic or administrative definitions. We used NCS-R data to estimate the prevalence of serious mental illness on the basis of recommendations from several researchers. In addition, the NCS-R was identified in a SAMHSA publication as a source of nationally representative data that measures the severity of mental disorders, which relates to SAMHSA's definition of serious mental illness.[73] Our draft clearly acknowledges the limitations of the NCS-R by stating that our estimate is likely to be low. It also provides the number of individuals 18 through 26 with serious mental illness who receive SSI and DI benefits due to mental illness. This number is likely to include young adults who may not have been included in the NCS-R, such as those living in an institution and many with schizophrenia or psychosis. To respond to HHS's comments, we have further highlighted our discussion of why limitations of the NCS-R result in an underestimate of the number of young adults with serious mental illness. With regard to the expertise of researchers and consumer organizations we interviewed, we chose the individuals and groups we did primarily because of their expertise in young adults with serious mental illness and, in many cases, because they were recommended to us by federal officials or researchers. While most also have an interest in a younger population, this group included organizations that have a strong interest in adult mental health issues, such as Mental Health America, several National Alliance of Mental Illness chapters, and Black Mental Health Alliance for Education and Consultation, Inc. In addition, we added information in response to HHS comments to better distinguish serious emotional disturbance from serious mental illness and information from other research on the degree to which state mental health agencies are implementing transition services.

As agreed with your offices, unless you make arrangements to release its contents earlier, we will make no further distribution of this report until 30 days from the date of this letter. At that time, we will send copies of this report to Education, DOJ, HHS, HUD, Labor, and SSA. Copies will also be made available to others on request. This report is also available at no charge on GAO's Web site at http://www.gao.gov.

Please contact us on (202) 512-7215 or (202) 512-7114 if you or your staff have any questions about this report. Contact points for our Office of Congressional Relations and Office of Public Affairs can be found on the last page of this report. Other major contributors to this report are listed in appendix XIV.

Cornelia M. Ashby
Director
Education, Workforce, and Income Security Issues

Cynthia A. Bascetta Director
Health Care Issues

In: Young Adults with Serious Mental Illness
Editor: David O. Sullivan
ISBN: 978-1-60692-641-3

APPENDIX I: SCOPE AND METHODOLOGY

To conduct our work, we relied on multiple methodologies, including data analyses, literature reviews, interviews, and site visits to four states. More specifically, to provide information on the number and demographic characteristics of young adults with serious mental illness, which we defined as individuals aged 18 through 26, we analyzed data from the federally funded National Comorbidity Survey-Replication, 200 1-2003 (NCS-R), of the 2006 Current Population Survey, Annual Social and Economic Supplement (CPS), and two sources of data on individuals receiving disability benefits from the Social Security Administration (SSA): the 2006 Ticket Research File (TRF) and the National Beneficiary Survey, 2004 (NBS). We also reviewed published research on the extent of mental illness among the homeless and those involved with the criminal justice or foster care systems. To identify the challenges faced by young adults with serious mental illness, we reviewed published research and interviewed federal, state, and local officials; mental health practitioners; experts; and advocacy groups. To describe the programs and strategies that selected states are using to assist these youth, we visited four states that had implemented programs specifically focused on this population— Connecticut, Maryland, Massachusetts, and Mississippi—and met with officials from key state agencies and private organizations involved in service delivery. To determine how federal agencies are supporting states and coordinating federal programs to help young adults with serious mental illness, we interviewed key federal officials from agencies within the U.S. Department of Education (Education), Department of Health and Human Services (HHS), Department of Housing and Urban Development (HUD), Department of Justice (DOJ), Department of Labor (Labor), and SSA. We also reviewed documents pertaining to the activities and accomplishments of interagency coordination groups, as well as funding and eligibility information on federal programs relevant to young adults with serious mental illness. We conducted our work from June 2007 through June 2008 in accordance with generally accepted government auditing standards.

DATA ANALYSES

To provide information on the number and demographic characteristics of young adults aged 18 through 26 with serious mental illness, we relied on data from the NCS-R, the CPS, the TRF, and the NBS. We considered using data from another survey, the National Survey on Drug Use and Health conducted by the Substance Abuse and Mental Health Services Administration (SAMHSA). Until 2004, SAMHSA reported rates of serious mental illness based on this survey but has since determined that the survey does not employ a sufficiently reliable measure of serious mental illness and therefore no longer uses it for this purpose.

The National Comorbidity Survey Replication

The NCS-R is a nationally representative survey of English-speaking household and campus group housing residents aged 18 and over living in the contiguous United States. Funded primarily by the National Institute of Mental Health, with supplemental funding from the National Institute on Drug Abuse and the Substance Abuse and Mental Health Services Administration (SAMHSA), the NCS-R served as the U.S. participation in the World Health Organization's World Mental Health Survey Initiative. The household sample was selected using a multistage clustered area probability sampling technique, and students living in campus-housing were selected from the household sample. Between February 2001 and April 2003, 7,693 individuals were interviewed, yielding a response rate of 71 percent. During the interviews, respondents were assessed for the presence of mental disorders within the previous year, using the Composite International Diagnostic Interview, a lay-administered survey that generates diagnoses based on the American Psychiatric Association's Diagnostic and Statistical Manual of Mental Disorders--Fourth Edition (DSM-IV) and the International Classification of Diseases--10.

To estimate the prevalence of serious mental illness in young adults, we obtained the NCS-R public use data file, as well as a supplemental file containing an indicator of the severity—serious, moderate, or mild—for each respondent diagnosed with a mental illness. This severity indicator was developed separately by the principal investigator of the NCS-R and is not included in the public use file. Using these two files, we isolated the 1,589 respondents who were aged 18 through 26 and identified the subset with serious mental illness[74] as well as the subset with moderate, mild, or no mental illness. We applied weighting variables to our estimates in order to project these results to the general population of young adults in the United States.[75] Following this methodology, we obtained a prevalence estimate of serious mental illness among young adults in U.S. households of 6.5 percent.

To estimate the total number of young adults with serious mental illness in 2006, we obtained population estimates from the 2006 CPS. We applied the 6.5 percent prevalence estimate to the total civilian, noninstitutionalized population estimate for young adults aged 18 through 26—37 million. Because NCS-R data pertain to individuals surveyed between February 2001 and April 2003, our 2006 estimates are based on the assumption that rates of serious mental illness were relatively stable among the young adult population from that survey period through 2006.[76] This is supported by research that shows that the prevalence of serious mental illness among adults in the United States did not change significantly between 1990 and 2003.

We also compared the demographic characteristics of the cohort of young adults aged 18 through 26 with serious mental illness to the cohort of young adults with mild or moderate mental illness and the cohort of those with no mental illness.[77] We applied weighting variables to project our results to the general population of young adults in the United States, and all estimates are presented using a 95 percent confidence interval, within plus or minus 12 percentage points, unless otherwise noted.[78] All tests of statistical significance were conducted at the 5 percent significance level for our analyses.

Ticket Research File

The TRF is a longitudinal database that combines administrative data from multiple SSA databases for all Supplemental Security Income (SSI) and Disability Insurance (DI) beneficiaries between age 18 and retirement age from 1996 through 2006. SSA provided us with an extract file containing data on the subset of 764,384 individuals aged 18 through 26 in 2006. We identified 186,101 individuals whose primary disability was listed as a serious mental illness at any point in 2006 by including those whose impairment fell under any of the following categories: major affective disorders, schizophrenia and psychoses, anxiety and neurotic disorders, and certain other mental disorders.[79] We then analyzed several characteristics of those individuals, including race, gender, primary and secondary disability, and benefit type, using information in the database.[80]

National Beneficiary Survey

Sponsored by SSA's Office of Disability and Income Security, the NBS is a nationally representative survey of SSI and DI beneficiaries and Ticket to Work participants between the ages of 18 and 64. The sample was selected using a multistage clustered sampling technique, and 6,520 individuals were interviewed between February and October 2004, for a weighted response rate of 77.5 percent. We used the same methodology for identifying the cohort of young adults with serious mental illness that we used for the TRF, based on each respondent's primary disabling condition. In total, the subsample contained 1,436 respondents aged 18 through 26 and 356 that were found to have a serious mental illness listed as their primary disability. We applied weighting variables to each estimate in order to project our results to the general population of young adults receiving disability benefits because of a serious mental illness, and all estimates are presented using a 95 percent confidence interval, within plus or minus 7 percentage points. Finally, we identified demographic data in the NBS that could be directly compared to demographic data in the NCS-R.

Data Reliability

We determined that data from the NCS-R, CPS, TRF, and NBS were sufficiently reliable for our purposes. In order to assess the reliability of the NCS-R, CPS, and NBS, we reviewed documentation pertaining to the sampling methodologies, survey instruments, and the structure of the data files. In order to assess the reliability of TRF data, we reviewed documentation on the construction of the file and the data reliability tests conducted by SSA's contractor—Mathematica Policy Research, Inc.

LITERATURE REVIEW

To provide information on the number of young adults with serious mental illness who are in certain vulnerable populations—specifically, those who are homeless or involved in the justice or foster care systems—we conducted a literature review that included published peer-reviewed research articles identified through databases such as ProQuest, Dissertations, Ovid, PsycINFO, PsycFirst, MEDLINE, ECO/WorldCat, Social Science Abstracts, and GAO publications. We used various search terms, such as young adult, mental illness, homeless, incarcerated, and foster care, in searching these databases, and we selected original research published since 1990. We were unable to identify any original research since 1990 that provided national estimates of the rates of serious mental illness in young adults in the three vulnerable populations. We did identify research on rates of mental illness in these vulnerable populations. We reviewed these studies' findings for methodological rigor and determined that they were sufficiently reliable for the purposes of this study.

To learn more about the major challenges faced by young adults with serious mental illness and their families, as well as their demographic characteristics, we conducted a literature review using the same databases identified above. We used various search terms, such as young adult, mental illness, challenges, support needs, service needs, family, and caregivers, and selected original research published since 1995. We also collected other literature cited in these studies as well as literature recommended to us during our interviews. We then conducted a more intensive review of the 18 studies identified through these methods. For each selected study, we reviewed the study's findings for methodological rigor and determined that it was sufficiently reliable for the purposes of this study.

Interviews with Researchers and Mental Health Organizations

To gather information related to all four objectives, we also conducted interviews with academic researchers and other experts on mental health issues, including some who represented mental health organizations. We identified interviewees through our literature review and through recommendations from federal agency officials and other mental health experts. In addition, we identified mental health-related organizations in the states we visited as part of our site visits. For this study we interviewed:

Hewitt B. Clark, Ph.D., University of South Florida; Maryann Davis, Ph. D., University of Massachusetts; Mary Molewyk Doornbos, Ph.D., R.N., Calvin College;

Donna Folkemer, National Conference of State Legislatures; Vicki Hines-Martin, Ph.D., R.N., C.S., University of Louisville;

Ronald C. Kessler, Ph.D., Harvard Medical School, Harvard University; Chris Koyanagi, Judge David L. Bazelon Center for Mental Health Law; Linda Rose, R.N., Ph.D., The Johns Hopkins University School of Nursing; Ann Vander Stoep, Ph.D., University of Washington;

Mary Wagner Ph.D., SRI International.

We also interviewed representatives from the following advocacy groups: Black Mental Health Alliance for Education and Consultation, Inc.; Maryland Coalition of Families for Children's Mental Health; Mississippi Families as Allies for Children's Mental Health, Inc.; Family Advocates for Children and Behavioral Health, Connecticut; National Federation of Families for Children's Mental Health; Generations United; National Alliance on Mental Illness, headquarters and chapters in Connecticut, Massachusetts, and Maryland; Mental Health America; National Family Caregivers Association; National Council on Independent Living; and Self Reliance, Inc., Center for Independent Living.

SITE VISITS

To describe the programs and strategies that selected states are using to assist young adults with serious mental illness, we visited four states that had implemented programs specifically focused on this population— Connecticut, Maryland, Massachusetts, and Mississippi. To identify these states, we reviewed published research and interviewed federal and state officials, mental health researchers, and advocacy groups to learn of states that were viewed as offering progressive statewide or state-organized programs that focus specifically on young adults with serious mental illness. Programs in these states should not be considered representative of how states assist young adults with serious mental illness nationally; rather, they serve as examples of states that are providing such assistance. We considered other states identified by research or by the officials, researchers, and advocacy groups, but these states generally had small, local programs available to serve young adults with serious mental illness, not statewide or state-organized programs. Before we made the site visits, we reviewed available literature on the four states' mental health systems and programs, including state mental health planning documents and federal grants pertaining to this population.

During the site visits, we met with officials from state mental health agencies, as well as other key state agencies and private sector organizations involved in providing, coordinating, or advocating for services for this population. During some of these meetings, we spoke with young adult consumers of state mental health services. Given that state mental health agencies are responsible for administering and coordinating services across the state for individuals with serious mental illness, we relied on each state mental health agency to serve as the lead agency in arranging visits with local mental health organizations, other state agencies, and private organizations.

While state programs that assist young adults with serious mental illness varied in the specific age ranges they targeted, for purposes of this report we focused on the key programs that state mental health agency officials identified, which generally served individuals aged 16 through 25. In addition, we reviewed written information on state policies and programs provided by state officials we interviewed.

In: Young Adults with Serious Mental Illness ISBN: 978-1-60692-641-3
Editor: David O. Sullivan

APPENDIX II: FEDERAL PROGRAMS IDENTIFIED BY BAZELON AS HELPING YOUNG ADULTS WITH A SERIOUS MENTAL ILLNESS (SMI)

Department	Program
Corporation for National and Community Service	Engaging Persons with Disabilities in National and Community Services Grants
DOJ	Drug-Free Communities Support Program Grants
	Juvenile Justice and Delinquency Prevention State Formula Grant
	Title V Community Prevention Grants Program
DOD	National Guard Youth ChalleNGe Program
Education	Elementary and Secondary School Counseling Program
	Federal Direct Student Loan and Family Education Loan Programs
	Grants for the Integration of Schools and Mental Health Systems
	Federal Perkins Loan Program
	Federal Supplemental Educational Opportunity Grants
	Federal Work-Study Program
	IDEA, Part B
	Independent Living Centers
	Pell Grants
	Safe and Drug Free Schools
	Transition Initiative
	Vocational and Adult Education State Basic Grants
	Vocational Rehabilitation: Supported Employment State Grants
	Vocational Rehabilitation, Title I Formula Grants
HHS	Adolescent Family Life Demonstration
	Child Care Block Grant
	Community Mental Health Services Block Grant
	Community Services Block Grant
	Comprehensive Community Mental Health Services for Children and Their Families

Appendix II (Continued).

Department	Program
	Educational and Training Vouchers Program for Youths Aging out of Foster Care
	Health Care for the Homeless
	Healthy and Ready to Work Initiative
	John H. Chafee Foster Care Independence Program
	Maternal & Child Health Block Grant
	Medicaid
	Partnerships for Youth in Transition
	Projects for Assistance in Transition from Homelessness - PATH
	Runaway and Homeless Youth Act Programs
	State Adolescent Substance Abuse Treatment Coordination
	S-CHIP
	Social Services Block Grant
	Substance Abuse Prevention and Treatment Block Grant
	Temporary Assistance for Needy Families
	Title IV-B and Promoting Safe and Stable Families
	Title IV-E – Payments for Children in Foster Care
	Youth Transition Into the Workplace Grant
HHS/Education/DOJ	Safe Schools and Healthy Students Initiative
	Community Development Block Grant
	HOME Investment Partnership
	Public Housing
	Section 8 Housing Choice Vouchers
	Shelter-Plus-Care
Labor	Job Corps
	One-Stop Career Centers
	Workforce Investment Act Youth Formula Grants
	YouthBuild
SSA	SSI Disability Benefits
	SSI Youth Transition Demonstration
	Ticket-To-Work and Work Incentives Improvement
USDA	Special Supplemental Nutrition for Women, Infants and Children (WIC)
	Food Stamps
	American Conservation and Youth Service Corps

Source: SAMHSA.

Note: On its website, SAMHSA provides toolkits for these five evidence-based practices. SAMHSA is also promoting and implementing research on evidence-based practices in a number of other areas, such as supportive housing and supported education, and plans on providing toolkits or other informational materials for these as well.

In: Young Adults with Serious Mental Illness
Editor: David O. Sullivan
ISBN: 978-1-60692-641-3

APPENDIX III: EVIDENCE-BASED PRACTICES PROMOTED BY SAMHSA

Evidence-Based Practice	Description
Assertive Community Treatment	Helps people stay out of the hospital and develop skills for living in the community, through treatment customized to individual needs delivered by a team of practitioners, available 24 hours a day.
Co-Occurring Disorders: Integrated Dual Disorders Treatment	Integrated treatment for mental illness and substance abuse addiction for people who have these co-occurring disorders.
Family Psychoeducation	Involves a partnership among consumers, families, and practitioners to learn ways to manage mental illness and reduce tension and stress within the family.
Illness Management and Recovery	Emphasizes helping people set and pursue personal goals and implement action strategies in their everyday lives.
Supported Employment	A well-defined approach to help people with mental illness find and keep competitive employment within their communities, through employment services that are integrated with mental health treatment.

Source: SAMHSA.

Note: On its website, SAMHSA provides toolkits for these five evidence-based practices. SAMHSA is also promoting and implementing research on evidence-based practices in a number of other areas, such as supportive housing and supported education, and plans on providing toolkits or other informational materials for these as well.

In: Young Adults with Serious Mental Illness ISBN: 978-1-60692-641-3
Editor: David O. Sullivan

APPENDIX IV: DEMOGRAPHIC CHARACTERISTICS OF YOUNG ADULTS AGED 18–26, BY SEVERITY OF MENTAL ILLNESS, 200 1–2003

Demographic characteristic		Serious mental illness	Moderate or mild mental illness	No mental illness
Sex	Male	45% (34-56)	43% (38-49)	53% (49-58)
	Female	55 (44-67)	57 (51-62)	47 (42-51)
Race	Caucasian	59 (47-72)	68 (61-75)	64 (59-70)
	African-American	19 (11-27)	11 (6-15)	12 (8-16)
	Hispanic	17 (10-24)	16 (11-21)	19 (15-23)
	Other	5 (1-8)	5 (2-9)	5 (3-7)
Region	Northeast	20 (11-28)	16 (11-21)	19 (12-27)
	Midwest	26 (17-36)	20 (15-26)	21 (17-26)
	South	34 (25-43)	35 (26-44)	33 (26-41)
	West	20 (8-32)	29 (16-41)	26 (15-37)
Marital status	Married	20 (13-28)	25.5 (21-30)	20 (16-23)
	Not married	80 (72-87)	74.5 (70-79)	80 (77-84)
Children	No children	71 (57-84)	75 (69-81)	81 (76-85)
	One child or more	29 (16-43)	25 (19-31)	19 (15-24)
Employment status	Employed	63 (52-75)	68 (62-73)	71 (67-75)
	Unemployed or student	37 (25-48)	32 (27-38)	29 (25-33)

Appendix IV (Continued).

Demographic characteristic		Serious mental illness	Moderate or mild mental illness	No mental illness
Education	0-11 years	36 (24-47)	19 (15-23)	17 (14-21)
	12 years	32 (24-40)	35 (28-42)	31 (25-38)
	More than 12 years	32 (24-41)	46 (39-54)	51 (44-59)
Health insurance	Insured	71 (61-81)	73 (38-78)	75 (70-80)
	Uninsured	29 (19-39)	27 (22-32)	25 (20-30)

Source: GAO analysis of the National Co-morbidity Survey Replication, 2001 -2003.
Note: Numbers in parentheses are confidence intervals at the 95% level.

In: Young Adults with Serious Mental Illness
Editor: David O. Sullivan
ISBN: 978-1-60692-641-3

APPENDIX V: DEMOGRAPHIC CHARACTERISTICS OF YOUNG ADULTS 18-26 WHO RECEIVED SSA DISABILITY BENEFITS BECAUSE OF A SMI

Demographic characteristic Results from the Ticket Research File, 2006		Among those with serious mental illness
Sex	Male	60%
	Female	40
Race	Caucasian	53
	African-American	29
	Hispanic	12
	Other or missing data	6
Benefit type	SSI payment	67
	DI payment	9
	Both	24
Results from the National Beneficiary Survey, 2004		
Marital status	Married	10% (6-13)
	Not married	90 (87-94)
Employment status	Employed	15 (10-19)
	Not employed	85 (81-90)
Ever worked	Yes	59 (53-66)
	No	41 (34-47)
Education	0–11 years	48 (41-55)

Appendix V: (Continued).

	12 years	42 (36-48)
Health insurance	More than 12 years	10 (7-13)
	Insured	93 (89-96)
	Uninsured	7 (4-11)

Source: GAO analysis of SSA's Ticket Research File, 2006, and National Beneficiary Survey, 2004.

Notes: This analysis does not include those who receive disability benefits because of abnormalities in cognition or intellectual functioning, such as mental retardation or autism. Numbers in parentheses are confidence intervals at the 95% level. Confidence intervals do not apply to statistics derived from the Ticket Research File, as they are true population values rather than estimates.

In: Young Adults with Serious Mental Illness
Editor: David O. Sullivan ISBN: 978-1-60692-641-3

APPENDIX VI: SELECTED PROGRAMS STATES CAN USE TO TARGET OR PROVIDE COMPREHENSIVE SERVICES FOR YOUNG ADULTS WITH SMI

Program	Department	Description
Justice and Mental Health Collaboration Program	DOJ	The Justice and Mental Health Collaboration Program was created to increase public safety by facilitating collaboration among the criminal justice, juvenile justice, and mental health and substance abuse treatment systems to increase access to services for offenders with mental illness.
Disability Program Navigator Initiative	Labor	Jointly funded by SSA and Labor, the Disability Program Navigator Initiative funds program liaisons who seek to coordinate all federally funded services to assist disabled individuals with employment training and employment placement at One-Stop centers which were established under the Workforce Investment Act of 1998.
Individuals with Disabilities Education Act Grants	Education	The Individuals with Disabilities Education Act authorizes formula grants to states and discretionary grants to institutions of higher education and other non-profit organizations to support research, demonstrations, technical assistance and dissemination, technology and personnel development, and parent-training and information centers.

(Continued).

Program	Department	Description
Vocational Rehabilitation Grants to States	Education	Under Title I of the Rehabilitation Act, these grants provide federal funds to help cover the costs of providing vocational rehabilitation services which include assessment, counseling, vocational and other training, and job placement necessary for an individual with a disability to achieve an employment outcome.
Rehabilitation Services Demonstration and Training Programs	Education	Activities under this program include carrying out special demonstrations for expanding and improving the provision of rehabilitation and other services including: technical assistance, special studies and evaluations, demonstrations of service delivery, transition services, supportive employment, services to underserved populations and/or unserved or underserved areas, among other services.
Mental Health Transformation State Incentive Grant	HHS	This SAMHSA grant focuses on a state's infrastructure in order to reduce fragmentation of services across systems.
Real Choice Systems Change Grants for Community Living	HHS	These CMS grants are specifically intended to help states build the infrastructure that will result in improvements in integrated community-based services.
Comprehensive Mental Health for Children and Families	HHS	This grant program was created by SAMHSA to provide community-based systems of care for children and adolescents with a serious emotional disturbance and their families.
Medicaid Buy-In	HHS	The CMS Medicaid buy-in program allows states to expand Medicaid coverage to workers with disabilities whose income and assets would ordinarily make them ineligible for Medicaid.
Medicaid Rehabilitation Option	HHS	The CMS Medicaid rehabilitation option provides a more flexible benefit and can be provided in other locations in the community, including in the person's home or other living arrangement. Rehabilitation services may extend beyond the clinical treatment of a person's mental illness to include helping the person to acquire the skills that are essential for everyday functioning.

Money Follows the Person	HHS	This grant creates a system of flexible financing for long-term services and supports that enable available funds to move with the individual to the most appropriate and preferred setting as the individual's needs and preferences change. Populations targeted for transition include individuals of all ages with disabilities including mental illness.

Source: GAO Analysis.

In: Young Adults with Serious Mental Illness
Editor: David O. Sullivan
ISBN: 978-1-60692-641-3

APPENDIX VII: OVERVIEW OF PROGRAMS FOR YOUNG ADULTS WITH SMI IN FOUR STATES

This appendix provides an overview of the key programs that target services for young adults with serious mental illness in the four states we visited—Connecticut, Maryland, Massachusetts, and Mississippi.

Connecticut's Department of Mental Health and Addiction Services administers the Young Adult Services program. Since 1998 in coordination with the Department of Children and Families and several other state agencies,[81] this program has provided mental health treatment, supported employment, vocational or educational support, life skills training, and supportive housing, with the particular array and level of care varying slightly by location.[82] Connecticut offers different levels of care, ranging from basic case management services and employment and educational support to highly structured group homes or supervised housing programs with intensive case management, or Assertive Community Treatment programs.[83] In addition, some programs are gender specific. Sixteen of the 21 local mental health authorities offer the Young Adult Services program. State officials indicated that they launched the program due to a federal lawsuit, which resulted in legislative funding for as special group of young adults who were diagnosed with pervasive developmental disorders and exhibited high risk sexual behavior issues. The program evolved to encompass a broader cohort of young adults with severe behavioral health issues and high risk behavior who, without any services, would have ended up in jail or homeless. Because many of these young adults spent most of their lives in institutional settings, such as psychiatric rehabilitative treatment centers, they had not developed interpersonal skills to effectively live in the community. In state fiscal year 2007, 716 individuals were served in the Young Adult Services program or about 27 percent of the 2,615 young adults with serious mental illness receiving any mental health services from the state mental health agency.

Maryland's Mental Hygiene Administration, within the Maryland Department of Health and Mental Hygiene, administers the Transition-Age Youth Initiative, which consists of various programs that provide mental health treatment, supported employment, life skills training, residential services, and, in some cases, supportive housing in the community. Eleven of the state's 20 mental health agencies offer services through this initiative, although the type and number of services offered vary by region. Some of these programs provide a greater array of services, including various types of mental health treatment services with supported employment, residential, and supportive housing, while others provide more limited case management services. Maryland mental health agency officials stated that program variety was beneficial, because a particular program design will work well for some young adults but not others. State officials told us that Maryland's Transition-Age Youth programs originated in the late 1990s when the Governor launched an initiative to expand services for young adults with disabilities who were transitioning from the children's system. As part of the initiative, funds were made available to the various agencies that serve these youth, including the Mental Hygiene Administration. With the money, mental health agency officials decided to fund a variety of types of small programs around the state, with the goal of evaluating them to identify promising programs that could be expanded. A Maryland mental health official said that funds were used to leverage and maximize other types of funds in order to create new services. While these Transition-Age Youth programs continue, a comprehensive evaluation has not been done. In fiscal year 2007, 8,753 young adults aged 18 through 24 received services from the Department of Mental Health and Hygiene, of which 415 received case management and 287 received supported employment services. In total, the state funded the Transition-Age Youth Initiative, which has capacity to treat about 250 individuals per year. Age criteria for individual programs differs, with one program serving individuals as young as 13 and another covering individuals as old as 25.

Massachusetts's Department of Mental Health established the Transition Age-Youth Initiative in 2005 to assist young adults with serious mental illness, including those transitioning from the children's mental health system to the adult system, as well as those aging out of foster care or the juvenile justice systems. This initiative provides an array of age- appropriate services to individuals aged 16 through 25 that address their needs in the areas of mental health treatment, vocational rehabilitation, employment, housing, peer support, and family psychoeducation. As part of this effort, as of January 2008, the Massachusetts Department of Mental Health had trained both child and adult case managers, as well as 36 Transition Age Youth case managers on the special needs of transition-age youth to better prepare them to assist young adults with serious mental illness in accessing services from the adult mental health system, according to a state mental health official. Transition-Age Youth services are available in all six Massachusetts Mental Health Service Delivery Areas, but the array of services differs by location. State officials cited several factors that influenced the development of the Transition-Age Youth Initiative. One factor was a concern about an area office that reported a decrease in the number of young adults requesting services after transitioning out of the children's mental health system. After researching the situation, the state found that the adult mental health program had not been providing the types of transition services that this age group needed and found appealing. Another factor was the issuance of the President's New Freedom Commission on Mental Health report and various other publications on transition-age youth by mental health researchers.[84] In 2007, about 2,600 individuals were enrolled in the Transition-Age Youth Initiative, according to a state mental health official.

In contrast with other states, Mississippi does not have a centralized and statewide program for young adults with serious mental illness but has several small-scale initiatives for this population. One of its key initiatives is the Transition Outreach Program, which provides mental health, supported employment, and life skills training to adolescents and young adults in two locations—Hattiesburg and Jackson. This program assists young adults in developing healthy relationships that can motivate them to change their behavior. This program developed because of the gap in services for the transition-age youth with serious mental illness. According to the officials, eventually young people would return to the mental health system, resurfacing at a mental health facility and in crisis. By June 2007, the Transitional Outreach Program had served more than 150 individuals. Another key initiative is the "Multidisciplinary Assessment and Planning Teams," which consist of officials from various state agencies and advocates that meet to review cases that include youth ages 14 to 21 transitioning from the child to adult mental health systems, as well as other youth considered to be high-risk. Established in 1996, these teams also coordinate the delivery of multiple services including mental health, education, vocational rehabilitation, health care, and juvenile justice services. As of November 2007 the teams were operating in 33 of 82 counties.

In: Young Adults with Serious Mental Illness ISBN: 978-1-60692-641-3
Editor: David O. Sullivan

APPENDIX VIII: COMMENTS FROM THE DEPARTMENT OF HEALTH AND HUMAN SERVICES

DEPARTMENT OF HEALTH & HUMAN SERVICES OFFICE OF THE SECRETARY

Assistant Secretary for Legislation
Washington, DC 20201

JUN 11 2008

Ms. Cornelia M. Ashby, Director
Education, Workforce, and
Income Security Issues
U.S. Government Accountability Office
441 G Street, NW
Washington, DC 20548

Dear Ms. Ashby:

Enclosed are the Department's comments on the U.S. Government Accountability Office's (GAO) draft report entitled: "Young Adults with Serious Mental Illness: Some States and Federal Agencies are Taking Steps to Address Their Challenges" (GAO 08-678).

The Department appreciates the opportunity to comment on this draft report before its publication.

Sincerely,

Vincent J. Ventimiglia, Jr.
Assistant Secretary for Legislation

Attachment

GENERAL COMMENTS OF THE DEPARTMENT OF HEALTH AND HUMAN SERVICES (HHS) ON THE GOVERNMENT ACCOUNTABILITY OFFICE'S (GAO) DRAFT REPORT ENTITLED: YOUNG ADULTS WITH SERIOUS MENTAL ILLNESS: SOME STATES AND FEDERAL AGENCIES ARE TAKING STEPS TO ADDRESS THEIR CHALLENGES (GAO-08-678)

HHS appreciates the opportunity to review this GAO report. This is a very pertinent and timely report, persons with some mental illnesses are diagnosed when they are children and transitioning to adulthood and aging out of certain systems can be a challenge for many.

The title may be more appropriately listed as **"Young Adults with Serious Mental Illness and Challenges in the Transition to Adulthood."** The current title seems to imply that the report will focus on all types of challenges, the most pertinent of which can include their actual symptoms, impairments, and the costs to the social support system.

Role of Families

The GAO has redefined the issues/questions and, therefore, has not answered two of the objectives "(1) *determine what is known about how many seriously mentally ill or seriously emotionally disturbed young adults are supported by their parents or grandparents and what are the key federal programs to assist them, and (2) determine if there are ways to reduce program overlap so that savings can be used to extend eligibility beyond age 18.*" There is almost no mention of families or the role that families can play in supporting young adults, an issue that is particularly important in the discussion of housing. For example, the data from the Clark County Washington Partnerships for Youth Transition (PYT) Grant showed that 60% of the youth were living at home with family members.

Program Overlap

Also GAO does not discuss ways to reduce program overlap which is critically important because funding defines policy and practice. If redundancies were to be identified that could be applied to this population, this report would provide an important contribution. One of the issues GAO highlights in the report is the narrower adult eligibility criteria for mental health services, and how that can eliminate receipt of needed services by individuals who have significant support needs but don't meet the stringent criteria. In a report sponsored by SAMHSA, Davis & Hunt (2005) state that adult mental health administrators identified lack of funding as one of the greatest barriers to improving services for young adults in their systems. Thus, the effort to identify such potential funds is critically important.

GENERAL COMMENTS OF THE DEPARTMENT OF HEALTH AND HUMAN SERVICES (HHS) ON THE GOVERNMENT ACCOUNTABILITY OFFICE'S (GAO) DRAFT REPORT ENTITLED: YOUNG ADULTS WITH SERIOUS MENTAL ILLNESS: SOME STATES AND FEDERAL AGENCIES ARE TAKING STEPS TO ADDRESS THEIR CHALLENGES (GAO-08-678)

Definition of Mental Illness

Also, the GAO needs to better define mental illness in this report. The GAO has not described the issue of Serious Emotional Disturbance (SED) vs. Serious Mental Illness (SMI), and has shifted to using ONLY the terminology of SMI. Furthermore, SMI is not well defined. The report describes the SAMHSA definition but doesn't use it in the analysis. Instead the report uses what is termed to be the DSM-IV's definition of mental illness. But DSM-IV doesn't define the term mental illness; it defines *mental disorder* which includes ALL disorders in the DSM-IV. The report then discounts cognitive disorders but not substance use disorders (both should not be included in any definition of mental illness). The report uses the NCS-R data to come up with a count, acknowledges that it didn't include homeless, institutionalized or incarcerated individuals, but doesn't mention that it didn't assess all diagnoses that could be considered either a mental illness by their definition or by SAMHSA's definition (the GAO excludes personality disorders because the NCS-R didn't assess it).

We suggest you list the definition as indicated by **Public Law 102-321** or consider using a term other than **"serious"** and defining exactly which disorders are classified using the new terminology. We are uncertain why **substance use disorders** would not fall into the category "serious mental illness."

- **Public Law 102-321** defines serious mental illness as the presence of any *Diagnostic and Statistical Manual of Mental Disorders* (DSM) mental disorder, substance use disorder, or developmental disorder that leads to "substantial interference" with "one or more major life activities." The diagnostic component of this definition was operationalized in the NCS with CIDI diagnoses of 3 broad classes of 12-month *DSM-III-R* disorders: mood disorders (major depression, dysthymia, bipolar disorder), anxiety disorders (panic disorder, generalized anxiety disorder, phobias, posttraumatic stress disorder), and nonaffective psychoses (schizophrenia, schizophreniform disorder, schizoaffective disorder, delusional disorder, brief psychotic disorder, and psychotic disorder not otherwise specified).

GENERAL COMMENTS OF THE DEPARTMENT OF HEALTH AND HUMAN SERVICES (HHS) ON THE GOVERNMENT ACCOUNTABILITY OFFICE'S (GAO) DRAFT REPORT ENTITLED: YOUNG ADULTS WITH SERIOUS MENTAL ILLNESS: SOME STATES AND FEDERAL AGENCIES ARE TAKING STEPS TO ADDRESS THEIR CHALLENGES (GAO-08-678)

Classification of the Population

Throughout the document, the GAO should specify whether the program/policy/research finding directly addresses this population or if only indirectly (e.g. all adults with SMI or all transition age youth with disabilities) so that it is clear to the reader what exactly that program/policy/research has to offer. The GAO should include some discussion about the issue of children being classified as having a SED and adults, at age 18 and older, being classified as having a SMI, and what that means. The report specifies it in the IDEA discussion, but not for mental health agency discussion (but use some studies of youths with SED). When the report uses more narrow/broad definitions, GAO should mention that the term used in childhood in mental health and education is "emotional disturbance", just to clarify that documents/programs/language that involves ED is related to this issue.

Estimates of Assistance or Support

In addition, the GAO was asked to provide "existing estimates of the number who do not receive the assistance or support they need." This is the crux of what is missing in this report. There is no estimate of unmet need and, therefore, no explanation of why there is unmet need. The report should address the fact that there is evidence (between their poor outcomes and the journal article Davis and Sondheimer published in 2006) that states do little in their adult mental health system to address the needs of this population, and why that is the case. Data in both that report and in a paper by Davis, Geller & Hunt, 2006, show that at least half of states adult mental health agencies were offering no programs tailored to this age group (as of 2003). In addition it is a difficult task for states to cobble together Federal programs that could address the needs of this population, and that those funds are currently used to address the needs of some other vulnerable group – so it means taking that away from that group in order to address the needs of this group – this is difficult for states to do without some encouragement and perhaps some incentives. Also the report to CMHS by Davis (Pioneering Transition Programs) highlights evidence that typical states struggle with how to address the needs of this population (and why) as well as the factors that administrators listed as problematic in addressing their needs.

GENERAL COMMENTS OF THE DEPARTMENT OF HEALTH AND HUMAN SERVICES (HHS) ON THE GOVERNMENT ACCOUNTABILITY OFFICE'S (GAO) DRAFT REPORT ENTITLED: YOUNG ADULTS WITH SERIOUS MENTAL ILLNESS: SOME STATES AND FEDERAL AGENCIES ARE TAKING STEPS TO ADDRESS THEIR CHALLENGES (GAO-08-678)

The GAO report should state that young adults are at the middle and end of a process of becoming an adult that starts before young adulthood in adolescence. Systems have organized themselves into child and adult and that has created a problem for young adults; they sometimes get dropped out and they often find programs that are not tailored to their needs because adult services are typically focused on full adulthood, not young adulthood. The GAO could clarify that some of the issues which arise from the transition age youth (TAY) literature (such as eligibility issues). Some of the issues raised in states regarding the young adult population directly stem from the recognition that some of the challenges start before adulthood. Some of the issues faced by young adults are defined by that immediately preceding period of life – as alluded to when describing eligibility and "transitional youth". GAO should acknowledge that improving services for transition age youth will, by definition, improve services for young adults and that several of the programs GAO reviewed are aimed at the transition period. Those typically are focused on individuals who were involved in systems or had illness as adolescents, and may not recognize newly ill young adults.

Tie Report Back to Original Concerns

Since the report offers concluding observations, the report should tie the findings back to the original concerns – that this population isn't finishing school (which should get them back to the transition issues), they aren't adequately employed, and they are arrested much more frequently. The report should acknowledge other research that has found other outcomes that is not adequately addressed with the NCS-R. When the GAO uses those findings to address outcomes it should be noted that those in the worst circumstances (e.g. those that adult MH should serve) would not have been picked up in the NCS-R.

Schizophrenia and Child-Serving Systems

The disjunction between the stated intent of the report and the findings presented, however, highlight the large gap that exists between child- and adult-serving systems of care in terms of populations served. Although the report mentions in several places that the service eligibility criteria for adults are narrower than those for children, nothing is said of the lack of experience and expertise in providing care for individuals with schizophrenia within child-serving systems.

GENERAL COMMENTS OF THE DEPARTMENT OF HEALTH AND HUMAN SERVICES (HHS) ON THE GOVERNMENT ACCOUNTABILITY OFFICE'S (GAO) DRAFT REPORT ENTITLED: YOUNG ADULTS WITH SERIOUS MENTAL ILLNESS: SOME STATES AND FEDERAL AGENCIES ARE TAKING STEPS TO ADDRESS THEIR CHALLENGES (GAO-08-678)

Analyses of Social Security disability data presented in the report reveal that schizophrenia is among the most prevalent diagnoses (33%) among adults with disabling mental illnesses. In contrast, schizophrenia is rare (4.7%) among those served by children's programs (Greenbaum et al., 1996). The discrepancy does not result from a difference in eligibility criteria but, rather, from the difference in the typical age of onset of the disorder.

Because schizophrenia typically emerges in the late teens or early adulthood, it is rarely seen in child-serving systems. Because the expertise in the treatment of schizophrenia primarily resides within adult-serving systems, young people with the disorder most often begin their course of treatment within the adult system, bypassing children's systems altogether. As the report correctly points out, although the adult system may have the best expertise for treating schizophrenia, it is not specifically designed to deal with young people and may hold little appeal to those seeking care.

Recognition of the difference in diagnoses served by the two systems is critical for ensuring that proposed solutions will adequately address the goals of transitional services. In the introductory sections of the report, GAO specifically mentions how difficult transition can be for young adults with schizophrenia. Yet, the methodology for reviewing programs that serve youth in transition is heavily weighted toward youth who were previously served by children's systems rather than those with newly emerging and debilitating illnesses in young adulthood. Indeed, the National Comorbidity Survey-Replication used to determine estimates of mental illness for this age group does not even include schizophrenia among diagnoses examined. The researchers and mental health organizations interviewed were heavily weighted to those with expertise in childhood illnesses and included neither experts in schizophrenia nor adult mental health primary consumer organizations.

In: Young Adults with Serious Mental Illness ISBN: 978-1-60692-641-3
Editor: David O. Sullivan

SELECTED BIBLIOGRAPHY

Bazelon Center for Mental Health Law. Moving On: Analysis of Federal Programs Funding Services to Assist Transition-Age Youth with Serious Mental Health Conditions. Washington, D.C.: 2005.

Burt, M., and others. Helping America's Homeless: Emergency Shelter or Affordable Housing? Washington, D.C.: Urban Institute Press, 2001.

Casey Family Programs. Improving Family Foster Care: Findings from the Northwest Foster Care Alumni Study. Seattle: 2005.

Clark, H. B., and others. "Partnerships for Youth Transition (PYT): Overview of Community Initiatives and Preliminary Findings on Transition to Adulthood for Youth and Young Adults with Mental Health Challenges," 329–32. In The 20th Annual Research Conference Proceedings: A System of Care for Children's Mental Health: Expanding the Research Base, edited by C. Newman and others. Tampa: University of South Florida, Louis de la Parte Florida Mental Health Institute, Research and Training Center for Children's Mental Health, 2008.

Clark, H. B., and others. "Services for Youth in Transition to Adulthood in Systems of Care." In The System of Care Handbook: Transforming Mental Health Services for Children, Youth, and Families, edited by B. A. Stroul and G. M. Blau. Baltimore: Paul H. Brookes, forthcoming.

Clark, H. B., and others. "Transition into Community Roles for Young People with Emotional or Behavioral Disorders: Collaborative Systems and Programs Outcomes." Chapter 11 in Transition of Secondary Students with Emotional or Behavioral Disorders: Current Approaches for Positive Outcomes, Arlington, Va.: *The Divisions of the Council for Exceptional Children,* 2004.

Consumer Quality Initiatives. Voices of Youth in Transition: The Experience of Aging Out of the Adolescent Public Mental Health Service System in Massachusetts: Policy Implications and Recommendations. *Dorchester, Mass.:* Dec. 11, 2002.

Davis, M., and others. "Longitudinal Patterns of Offending During the Transition to Adulthood in Youth from the Mental Health System." *The Journal of Behavioral Health Services and Research.* 31, no. 4 (2004): 351–66.

Davis, M., J. Geller, and B. Hunt. "Within-State Availability of Transition-to-Adulthood Services for Youths with Serious Mental Health Conditions." *Psychiatric Services.* 57, no. 11 (2006): 1594–99.

Davis, Maryann. "Improving Youth Transitions Systems and Measuring Change." Paper, National Partnerships for Youth in Transition Forum, Center for Mental Health Services, Massachusetts, August, 2005.

Davis, Maryann. Pioneering Transition Programs: The Establishment of Programs That Span the Ages Served by Child and Adult Mental Health. Rockville, Md.: Substance Abuse and Mental Health Services Administration, Center for Mental Health Services, 2007.

Davis, Maryann, and Nancy Koroloff. "The Great Divide: How Mental Health Policy Fails Young Adults" *Research in Community and Mental Health.* 14 (2006): 53–74.

Davis, Maryann, and Diane L. Sondheimer. "State Child Mental Health Efforts to Support Youth in Transition to Adulthood." *Journal of Behavioral Health Services and Research.* 32, no. 1 (2005): 27–42.

Davis, Maryann, and Ann Vander Stoep. The Transition to Adulthood among Adolescents Who Have Serious Emotional Disturbance. Prepared for The Delmar, New York, National Resource Center on Homelessness and Mental Illness Policy Research Associates. Rockville, Md.: Center for Mental Health Services, Substance Abuse and Mental Health Services Administration, April 1996.

Deschenes, N., H. B. Clark, and J. Herrygers. "Evaluating Fidelity of Community Programs for Transition-Age Youth," 137–39. In The 21st Annual Research Conference Proceedings: A System of Care for Children's Mental Health: Expanding the Research Base, edited by C. Newman and others. Tampa: University of South Florida. Louis de la Parte Florida Mental Health Institute, *Research and Training Center for Children's Mental Health,* 2008.

Doornbos, Mary Molewyk. "The 24-7-52 Job: Family Caregiving for Young Adults with Serious and Persistent Mental Illness." *Journal of Family Nursing.* 7, no. 4 (2001): 328–44

Doornbos, Mary Molewyk. "Family Caregivers and the Mental Health Care System: Reality and Dreams." *Archives of Psychiatric Nursing.* 16, no. 1 (2002): 39–46.

Greenbaum, P. E., and others. "National Adolescent and Child Treatment Study (NACTS): Outcomes for Children with Serious Emotional and Behavioral Disturbance." *Journal of Emotional and Behavioral Disorders.* 4, no. 3 (1996): 130–46.

Haber, M. G., and others. "Predicting Improvement of Transitioning Young People in the Partnerships for Youth Transition Initiative: Findings from a Multi-Site Demonstration." *Journal of Behavioral Health Services and Research, forthcoming.*

Hines-Martin, V., and others. "Barriers to Mental Health Care Access in an African American Population." *Issues in Mental Health Nursing.* 24 (2003): 237–56.

Hines-Martin, Vicki P. "Environmental Context of Caregiving for Severely Mentally Ill Adults: An African American Experience." *Issues in Mental Health Nursing.* 19 (1998): 433–51.

Horwitz, Allan V. and Susan C. Reinhard. "Ethnic Differences in Caregiving Duties and Burdens among Parents and Siblings of Persons with Severe Mental Illnesses." *Journal of Health and Social Behavior.* 36, no. 2 (1995): 138–50.

James, D. and L. Glaze. Mental Health Problems of Prison and Jail Inmates. Special report prepared by the Bureau of Justice Statistics, U.S. Department of Justice. Washington, D.C.: 2006.

Johnson, Eric D. "Differences among Families Coping with Serious Mental Illness: A Qualitative Analysis." *American Journal of Orthopsychiatry.* 70, no. 1 (2000): 126–34.

Karpur, A. H. B. Clark, P. Caproni, and H. Sterner. "Transition to Adult Roles for Students with Emotional/Behavioral Disturbances: A Follow-Up Study of Student Exiters from Steps-to-Success." *Career Development for Exceptional Individuals.* 28, no. 1 (2005): 36–46.

Kaye, Steve. Employment and Social Participation among People with Mental Health Disabilities. San Francisco: National Disability Statistics and Policy Forum, 2002.

Kessler, R., and others. "The Prevalence and Correlates of Serious Mental Illness (SMI) in the National Comorbidity Survey Replication (NCS-R)." In Mental Health, United States, 2004, edited by R. W. Manderscheid and J.

T. Berry. DHHS Publication (SMA)-06-4195. Rockville, Md.: Substance Abuse and Mental Health Services Administration, 2006.

Kessler, R., and others. "Prevalence, Severity, and Comorbidity of 12- Month DSM-IV Disorders in the National Comorbidity Survey Replication." *Archives of General Psychiatry*. 62 (2005): 6 17–27.

Kessler, R., and others. "Prevalence and Treatment of Mental Disorders, 1990 to 2003." *The New England Journal of Medicine*. 352, no. 24 (2005): 2515–23.

Mays, Gloria D. and Carole L. Lund. "Male Caregivers of Mentally Ill Relatives." *Perspectives in Psychiatric Care*. 35, no. 2 (1999): 19–28.

National Collaborative on Workforce and Disability for Youth, Institute for Educational Leadership. Tunnels & Cliffs: A Guide for Workforce Development Practitioners and Policymakers Serving Youth with Mental Health Needs. Number E-9-4-1-0070. Washington, D.C.: March 2007.

New Freedom Commission on Mental Health. Achieving the Promise: Transforming Mental Health Care in America: Final Report. DHHS Publication SMA-03-3832. Rockville, Md.: 2003.

Pilowsky, Daniel J. and Li-Tzy Wu. "Psychiatric Symptoms and Substance Use Disorders in a Nationally Representative Sample of American Adolescents Involved with Foster Care." *Journal of Adolescent Health*. 38 (2006): 351–58.

Rose, L., R. K. Mallinson and L. D. Gerson. "Mastery, Burden, and Areas of Concern among Family Caregivers of Mentally Ill Persons." *Archives of Psychiatric Nursing*. 20, no. 1 (2006): 4 1–51.

Rose, Linda. "Caring for Caregivers: Perceptions of Social Support." *Journal of Psychosocial Nursing and Mental Health Services*. 35, no. 2 (1997): 17–24.

Shufelt, Jennie L. and Joseph J. Cocozza. Youth with Mental Health Disorders in the Juvenile Justice System: Results from a Multi-State Prevalence Study. Delmar, N.Y.: National Center for Mental Health and Juvenile Justice, 2006.

Smiley, Amy, and Alysia Pascaris. A Chance for Change: Supporting Youth in Transition in New York City: A Report on the Findings of the 2006–2007 Youth Initiative Work Group. New York: Coalition of Behavioral Health Agencies, 2007.

Styron, T. H., and others. "Troubled Youth in Transition: An Evaluation of Connecticut's Special Services for Individuals Aging Out of Adolescent Mental Health Programs." *Children and Youth Services Review*. 28, no. 9 (2006): 1088–101.

Unger, J., and others. "Homeless Youths and Young Adults in Los Angeles: Prevalence of Mental Health Problems and the Relationship between Mental Health and Substance Abuse Disorders." *American Journal of Community Psychology*. 25 (1997): 371–94.

Vander Stoep, Ann. "Through the Cracks: Transition to Adulthood for Severely Psychiatrically Impaired Youth," 357–68. In The 4th Annual Research Conference Proceedings, A System of Care for Children's Mental Health: Expanding the Research Base, edited by A. Algarin and R. Friedman. Tampa: University of South Florida, Florida Mental Health Institute, *Research and Training Center for Children's Mental Health,* 1992.

Wagner, Mary M. "Outcomes for Youths with Serious Emotional Disturbance in Secondary School and Early Adulthood." *The Future of Children.* 5, no. 2 (1995): 90-112.

Wagner, Mary and Maryann Davis. "How Are We Preparing Students with Emotional Disturbances for the Transition to Young Adulthood? Findings from the National Longitudinal Transition Study—2." *Journal of Emotional and Behavioral Disorders.* 14, no. 2 (2006): 86–98.

In: Young Adults with Serious Mental Illness
Editor: David O. Sullivan
ISBN: 978-1-60692-641-3

RELATED GAO PRODUCTS

GAO, Disconnected Youth: Federal Action Could Address Some of the Challenges Faced by Local Programs That Reconnect Youth to Education and Employment, GAO-08-313 (Washington, D.C.: Feb. 28, 2008)

GAO, Residential Treatment Programs: Concerns Regarding Abuse and Death in Certain Programs for Troubled Youth, GAO-08-146T (Washington, D.C.: Oct. 10, 2007)

GAO, School Mental Health: Role of the Substance Abuse and Mental Health Services Administration and Factors Affecting Service Provision, GAO-08-19R (Washington, D.C.: Oct. 05, 2007)

GAO, Child Welfare: HHS Actions Would Help States Prepare Youth in the Foster Care System for Independent Living, GAO-07-1097T (Washington, D.C.: Jul. 12, 2007)

GAO, African American Children in Foster Care: Additional HHS Assistance Needed to Help States Reduce the Proportion in Care, GAO-07- 816 (Washington, D.C.: Jul. 11, 2007)

GAO, Child Welfare: Additional Federal Action Could Help States Address Challenges in Providing Services to Children and Families, GAO-07-850T (Washington, D.C.: May. 15, 2007)

GAO, Child Welfare: Improving Social Service Program, Training, and Technical Assistance Information Would Help Address Long-standing Service-Level and Workforce Challenges, GAO-07-75 (Washington, D.C.: Oct. 06, 2006)

GAO, D.C. Child and Family Services Agency: Performance Has Improved, but Exploring Health Care Options and Providing Specialized Training May Further Enhance Performance, GAO-06-1093 (Washington, D.C.: Sep. 28, 2006)

GAO, Summary of a GAO Conference: Helping California Youths with Disabilities Transition to Work or Postsecondary Education, GAO-06- 759SP (Washington, D.C.: Jun. 20, 2006)

GAO, Child Welfare: Federal Oversight of State IV-B Activities Could Inform Action Needed to Improve Services to Families and Statutory Compliance, GAO-06-787T (Washington, D.C.: May. 23, 2006)

GAO, Children's Health Insurance: Recent HHS-OIG Reviews Inform the Congress on Improper Enrollment and Reductions in Low-Income, Uninsured Children, GAO-06-457R (Washington, D.C.: Mar. 09, 2006)

GAO, District of Columbia: Federal Funds for Foster Care Improvements Used to Implement New Programs, but Challenges Remain, GAO-05-787 (Washington, D.C.: Jul. 22, 2005)

GAO, Medicaid Financing: States' Use of Contingency-Fee Consultants to Maximize Federal Reimbursements Highlights Need for Improved Federal Oversight, GAO-05-748, (Washington, D.C.: June 28, 2005).

GAO, Child Welfare: Better Data and Evaluations Could Improve Processes and Programs for Adopting Children with Special Needs, GAO- 05-292 (Washington, D.C.: Jun. 13, 2005)

GAO, Medicaid Managed Care: Access and Quality Requirements Specific to Low-Income and Other Special Needs Enrollees, GAO-05-44R (Washington, D.C.: Dec. 08, 2004)

GAO, Foster Youth: HHS Actions Could Improve Coordination of Services and Monitoring of States' Independent Living Programs, GAO- 05-25 (Washington, D.C.: Nov. 18, 2004)

GAO, D.C. Child And Family Services Agency: More Focus Needed on Human Capital Management Issues for Caseworkers and Foster Parent Recruitment and Retention, GAO-04-1017 (Washington, D.C.: Sep. 24, 2004)

GAO, Substance Abuse and Mental Health Services Administration: Planning for Program Changes and Future Workforce Needs is Incomplete, GAO-04-683 (Washington, D.C.: June 4, 2004)

GAO, Child Welfare: Improved Federal Oversight Could Assist States in Overcoming Key Challenges, GAO-04-418T (Washington, D.C.: Jan. 28, 2004)

GAO, Child Welfare: Enhanced Federal Oversight of Title IV-B Could Provide States Additional Information to Improve Services, GAO-03-956 (Washington, D.C.: Sep. 12, 2003)

GAO, Child Welfare: Most States Are Developing Statewide Information Systems, but the Reliability of Child Welfare Data Could Be Improved, GAO-03-809 (Washington, D.C.: Jul. 31, 2003)

GAO, Child Welfare and Juvenile Justice: Several Factors Influence the Placement of Children Solely to Obtain Mental Health Services, GAO-03-865T (Washington, D.C.: Jul. 17, 2003)

GAO, Child Welfare and Juvenile Justice: Federal Agencies Could Play a Stronger Role in Helping States Reduce the Number of Children Placed Solely to Obtain Mental Health Services, GAO-03-397 (Washington, D.C.: Apr. 21, 2003)

GAO, Medicaid and SCHIP: States Use Varying Approaches to Monitor Children's Access to Care, GAO-03-222 (Washington, D.C.: Jan. 14, 2003)

REFERENCES

[1] For purposes of this report, the term "mental illness" excludes mental disorders that constitute abnormalities in cognition or intellectual functioning, such as mental retardation, autism, or Alzheimer's disease.

[2] All NCS-R and NBS estimates of the number and demographic characteristics of young adults with serious mental illness are presented with a 95 percent confidence interval. Unless otherwise noted, the sampling error is within plus or minus 12 percentage points for NCS-R estimates and within plus or minus 7 percentage points for NBS estimates.

[3] These states are not considered representative of all states in the manner and extent to which they assist young adults with serious mental illness.

[4] In this report, transition-aged youth programs generally refer to programs that include individuals aged 16 through 25, although programs vary with some serving a broader age range.

[5] Mental disorders are diagnosed using criteria in the Diagnostic and Statistical Manual of Mental Disorders--Fourth Edition (DSM-IV). Each diagnosis, such as generalized anxiety disorder, major depressive disorder, or schizophrenia, is based on a specific set of symptoms reported over a given period of time. For example, major depressive disorder can be diagnosed if an individual reports experiencing five or more of seven specified symptoms, such as fatigue, feelings of worthlessness or excessive or inappropriate guilt, and a diminished ability to concentrate, over a minimum of 2 weeks.

[6] Those with mental health issues in childhood may be considered to have a "serious emotional disturbance" defined as "persons from birth up to age 18, who currently or at any time during the past year, have

had a diagnosable mental, behavioral, or emotional disorder of sufficient duration to meet diagnostic criteria specified within DSM-III-R, that resulted in functional impairment which substantially interferes with or limits the child's role or functioning in family, school, or community activities." 58 *Fed. Reg.* 29422 (May 20, 1993). The DSM-III-R predates the DSM-IV.

[7] Kessler, R., P. Berglund, O. Demler, R. Jin, K. Merikangas, and E. Walters. "Lifetime Prevalence and Age-of-Onset Distributions of DSM-IV Disorders in the National Comorbidity Survey Replication." Archives of General Psychiatry 62 (2005): 593-602.

[8] Pub. L. No. 102-321, § 201. Mental Health Block Grant funding is also targeted to children with a serious emotional disturbance.

[9] 58 *Fed. Reg.* 29422 (May 20, 1993). This report generally uses the term "serious mental illness" based on SAMHSA's regulation. However, in places throughout this report, we may use a slightly broader or narrower conception of serious mental illness as necessitated by available data as well as programmatic or administrative definitions.

[10] Individuals can also qualify if they can demonstrate that they have a physical impairment that is expected to result in death.

[11] Individuals known as "disabled adult children" can also receive DI benefits if they are aged 18 or older, were disabled before age 22, and have at least one parent who also receives Social Security payments because of retirement or disability or who is deceased but worked long enough to be eligible to receive benefits.

[12] In most states, individuals receiving SSI are also eligible for Medicaid.

[13] The Medicaid rehabilitation option provides a more flexible benefit and can be provided in other locations in the community, including in the person's home or other living arrangement. Rehabilitation services may extend beyond the clinical treatment of a person's mental illness to include helping the person to acquire the skills that are essential for everyday functioning. For GAO work that addresses the rehabilitation option, see *Medicaid Financing: States' Use of Contingency-Fee Consultants to Maximize Federal Reimbursements Highlights Need for Improved Federal Oversight,* GAO-05-748 (Washington, D.C.: June 28, 2005).

[14] According to SAMHSA, these evidence-based practices have been tested on the adult population, which included some young adults aged 18 through 30, but have not been systematically or empirically tested specifically on the young adult population.

[15] For a GAO study related to SAMHSA's administration of mental health programs, see Substance Abuse and Mental Health Services Administration: Planning for Program Changes and Future Workforce Needs Is Incomplete, GAO-04-683 (Washington, D.C.: June 4, 2004).

[16] As defined by the Individuals with Disabilities Education Act, an emotional disturbance is a condition exhibiting certain characteristics over a long period of time and to a marked degree that adversely affects educational performance. The characteristics include an inability to learn that cannot be explained by intellectual, sensory, or health factors and inappropriate types of behavior or feelings under normal circumstances, among others.

[17] The Foster Care Independence Act also authorizes $60 million for payments to states for postsecondary educational and training vouchers for youth likely to experience difficulty as they transition to adulthood after the age of 18.

[18] See GAO, Child Welfare: HHS Actions Would Help States Prepare Youth in the Foster Care System for Independent Living, GAO-07-1097T (Washington, D.C.: July 12, 2007).

[19] The sampling error for this estimate is plus or minus 1.2 percentage points.

[20] While estimates of the size of these populations exist, they are for different years and are not all recent. The National Survey of Homeless Assistance Providers and Clients estimated that between 124,000 and 236,000 individuals aged 20 through 24 were homeless in 1996. According to Bureau of Justice Statistics officials, about 222,000 young adults aged 18 through 24 were incarcerated in federal or state prison in 2004, and about 177,000 were in local jails in 2002. While the total number of institutionalized young adults is unknown, one study found that the average number of individuals who were institutionalized because of a mental illness on any day in 1992 was nearly 84,000.

[21] Prevalence estimates may also be affected by the exclusion of non-English-speaking households from the survey.

[22] Schizophrenia and nonaffective psychosis are characterized by an inability to distinguish between what is real and what is imaginary. Symptoms include delusions, hallucinations, extreme apathy, and social withdrawal. According to NCS-R researchers, household surveys may underestimate the prevalence of these disorders, because these individuals may be less likely than those with other types of serious mental illness to live at home or be less willing to participate in a

survey. However, to the extent that they do live at home, researchers believe they are likely to be represented in the NCS-R estimates because many are diagnosed with multiple mental disorders.

[23] The NCS-R provides separate prevalence estimates for bipolar I and bipolar II disorder. For the purposes of this analysis, we add the estimates together to derive the prevalence of bipolar disorder generally.

[24] The NCS-R does not distinguish between primary and secondary diagnoses.

[25] The sampling error for this estimate is plus or minus 13 percentage points. Drug abuse, drug dependence, alcohol abuse, and alcohol dependence are all considered diagnosable mental illnesses in the DSM-IV. In general, substance abuse is defined as the continued use of a substance despite school-related or work-related or interpersonal problems. Dependence is characterized by an increasing need for the substance to achieve the desired effects as well as withdrawal symptoms when the substance is not used.

[26] Steve Kaye. *Employment and Social Participation among People with Mental Health Disabilities.* (San Francisco: National Disability Statistics and Policy Forum, 2002).

[27] The President's New Freedom Commission on Mental Health, *Achieving the Promise: Transforming Mental Health Care in America: Final Report*, DHHS Publication SMA-03- 3832 (Rockville, Md.: 2003).

[28] Individuals are not eligible to receive SSI or DI benefits for a drug or alcohol addiction that is material to the disability determination; however, some individuals with a substance-related disorder may be eligible because of another disability.

[29] Those receiving SSI or DI are encouraged to participate in the Ticket to Work program, an employment program administered by SSA that provides rehabilitation opportunities and support for disabled individuals to return to work without automatically losing their cash benefits and health care coverage.

[30] As a result, many people may need another adult's help when applying for or while receiving benefits. In fact, nearly 68 percent of SSI recipients with a serious mental illness in 2006 had a representative payee who received the payments on their behalf, and just over half of these payees were parents or other relatives.

[31] Secondary diagnosis is defined as the most significant diagnosis in terms of severity following the primary diagnosis.

[32] D. Pilowsky and L.T. Wu, "Psychiatric Symptoms and Substance Use Disorders in a Nationally Representative Sample of American Adolescents Involved with Foster Care," *Journal of Adolescent Health* 38 (2006): 35 1-58.

[33] See Casey Family Programs, Improving Family Foster Care: Findings from the Northwest Foster Care Alumni Study (Seattle, WA: 2005).

[34] In this study, respondents were classified as having a mental health problem if they met one of several conditions—for example, if they reported that they had been receiving treatment or been hospitalized for mental or emotional problems or if they reported that a mental health condition was the single largest factor keeping them from getting out of homelessness. See M. Burt and others, *Helping America's Homeless: Emergency Shelter or Affordable Housing?* (Washington, D.C.: Urban Institute Press, 2001) 157.

[35] J. Unger and others, "Homeless Youths and Young Adults in Los Angeles: Prevalence of Mental Health Problems and the Relationship between Mental Health and Substance Abuse Disorders," *American Journal of Community Psychology* 25 (1997): 371-94.

[36] In this study, respondents were classified as having a mental health problem using two measures: a recent history or symptoms of a mental health problem within the past 12 months. A recent history included a clinical diagnosis or treatment by a mental health professional. Symptoms of a mental disorder were based on criteria specified in the DSMIV. See James, Doris J. and Glaze, Lauren E. *Mental Health Problems of Prison and Jail Inmates*, a special report prepared by the Bureau of Justice Statistics, September 2006.

[37] Mental health disorders were identified using the Diagnostic Interview Schedule for Children—Voice Version IV, a structured interview designed to measure over 30 psychiatric diagnoses common among adolescents. Severe mental illnesses were those that met criteria for certain severe disorders that required significant or immediate treatment or resulted in hospitalization. See Jennie L. Shufelt and Joseph J. Cocozza, *Youth with Mental Health Disorders in the Juvenile Justice System: Results from a Multi-State Prevalence Study* (Delmar, N.Y.: National Center for Mental Health and Juvenile Justice, 2006).

[38] GAO, Disconnected Youth: Federal Action Could Address Some of the Challenges Faced by Local Programs That Reconnect Youth to Education and Employment, GAO-08-313 (Washington, D.C.: Feb. 28, 2008).

[39] Consumer Quality Initiatives, Voices of Youth in Transition Report the Experience of Aging Out of the Adolescent Public Mental Health Service System in Massachusetts: Policy Implications and Recommendation (Dorchester, Mass.: Dec. 11, 2002).

[40] Several mental health advocates have noted that it may also be difficult for young adults to find culturally competent or linguistically appropriate mental health care. The Surgeon General noted in the 2001 report - *Mental Health: Culture, Race, and Ethnicity – A Supplement to Mental Health: A Report of the Surgeon General* – that racial and ethnic minorities have less access to mental health services and are less likely to receive needed care.

[41] While vocational rehabilitation programs have been traditionally used by those with physical, more than half of all persons who exit these with an employment outcome have some type of mental impairment, broadly defined. Within that broad category, in FY 2006, persons with mental illness specifically comprised 31 percent of all vocational rehabilitation applicants and represented 23 percent of all consumers who exited with an employment outcome.

[42] SAMHSA is beginning to develop a resource guide on supported education which is intended to help individuals with serious mental illness begin or return to postsecondary education.

[43] SAMSHA, *What a Difference a Friend Makes: Social Acceptance Is Key to Mental Health Recovery,* National Mental Health Anti-Stigma Campaign, SMA 07-4257 (Washington, D.C.: March 2007) http://mentalhealth.samhsa.gov/publications/allpubs/SMA07-4257/default.asp.

[44] National Conference of State Legislatures, A Difficult Passage: Helping Youth with Mental Health Needs Transition into Adulthood, Michelle Herman, (September 2006).

[45] Maryann Davis and Nancy Koroloff, "The Great Divide: How Mental Health Policy Fails Young Adults," *Research in Community and Mental Health* 14: 53–74.

[46] However, SSA officials noted that adults may be deemed eligible for SSI or DI based on symptoms related to a disorder that qualified them as children, even if the disorder itself did not.

[47] National Collaborative on Workforce and Disability for Youth, Institute for Educational Leadership. *Tunnels and Cliffs: A Guide for Workforce Development Practitioners and Policymakers Serving Youth with Mental Health Needs,* Office of Disability Employment Policy E-9-4-1-0070 (Washington, D.C.: March 2007).

[48] Judge David L. Bazelon Center for Mental Health Law, Moving On: Analysis of Federal Programs Funding Services to Assist Transition-Age Youth with Serious Mental Health Conditions (Washington, D.C.: 2005).

[49] With regard to states in general, research based on 2003 survey data from 41 states and the District of Columbia found that one half of state adult mental health systems offered some transition services, but few provided any kind of transition service at more than one site. See Davis, M., J. Geller, and B. Hunt. "Within-State Availability of Transition-to-Adulthood Services for Youths with Serious Mental Health Conditions" Psychiatric Services 57, no. 11 (2006): 1594-1599.

[50] State officials noted that their programs are culturally competent because they take into account a participant's age, race, gender, and culture.

[51] Connecticut's Department of Children and Families is responsible for providing children and adolescents' behavioral health services, juvenile justice and protection services.

[52] Individuals receiving Assertive Community Treatment services have a variety of mental health impairments, such as difficulties with basic, everyday activities like keeping themselves safe, caring for their basic physical needs, or maintaining safe and adequate housing. They may also struggle with unemployment, substance abuse, homelessness, and involvement in the criminal justice system.

[53] Assertive Community Treatment team members are cross-trained in each other's areas of expertise to the maximum extent feasible. The team, which typically works with a relatively small number of individuals, is available for support as long as the services are needed.

[54] All 30 evidence-based programs can serve young adults, but six of these are separate programs specifically designed for young adults aged 17 and above.

[55] The supported education counselor works closely with the state adult and child mental health agencies and with youth formerly in foster care or juvenile justice who are transitioning out of the child mental health system.

[56] In addition to mental health agency officials, the Task Force consists of officials from Mississippi's Department of Rehabilitation Services; Department of Human Services (foster care); Mississippi Families as Allies, a nonprofit advocacy organization for individuals with mental illnesses and their families; and senior program staff from the Transitional Outreach Program. This task force meets twice a year.

[57] Maryland also uses a team approach in local jurisdictions to address transition issues of young adults receiving residential services.

[58] Other health care services that can be provided under this option include other diagnostic, screening, preventive, and rehabilitation services and certain evidence-based practices such as Assertive Community Treatment.

[59] Connecticut mental health officials told us that they have chosen not to use the rehabilitation option to cover services associated with the state's program for young adults with serious mental illness, but they use it to cover other mental health services.

[60] Person-centered planning is an approach that emphasizes individualized services and consumer choice in treatment.

[61] Some state mental health agencies provided grants to nonprofit agencies that administer their young adult program to help pay for services not covered by Medicaid.

[62] The Housing Choice Voucher program is authorized by section 8 of the U.S. Housing Act of 1937, as amended (42 U.S.C. 1437f). Regulations are found in 24 C.F.R. Part 982. HUD's Office of Public and Indian Housing oversees the administration of the program.

[63] Local public housing agencies administer the Section 8 Housing Choice Voucher program on HUD's behalf and provide eligible households with a subsidy to seek and rent suitable housing in the private market. These vouchers can be used in group homes for persons with serious mental illness.

[64] One-Stop Centers provide employment training and placement to any individual seeking work.

[65] The TIP System model is driven by seven guidelines or principles that include but are not limited to engaging young people through relationship development and person-centered planning, providing developmentally appropriate services and supports, and teaching life-skills. The model can be used as part of case management or in a team format, such as Assertive Community Treatment. The TIP system is based on research that includes outcomes. According to its author, the

TIP model is an "evidence-supported practice" based on the findings from numerous outcomes studies. However, it has not been evaluated against a control group using random clinical assignment. For details regarding the TIP model, see http://tip.fmhi.usf.edu and Clark, H. B. *Transition to Independence Process System Development and Operations Manual* University of South Florida (Florida) *2004.*

[66] In 2002, two executive orders highlighted issues concerning fragmentation across mental health and youth-serving programs. These executive orders created the President's New Freedom Commission on Mental Health and the White House Task Force on Disadvantaged Youth.

[67] The grant also funded services for youth with serious emotional disturbances.

[68] It should be noted that this evaluation lacked a control group and, according to the researchers, improvements identified might be explained by factors other than the program, such as attrition and maturation effects, despite efforts to account for such factors in their analyses. Also, the results are limited to the 193 program participants for whom data were available and should be not generalized to all program participants. M.G. Haber and others, "Predicting Improvement of Transitioning Young People in the Partnerships for Youth Transition Initiative: Findings from a Multi-Site Demonstration," *Journal of Behavioral Health Services and Research*, forthcoming.

[69] National Collaborative on Workforce & Disability for Youth, Institute for Educational Leadership, *Tunnels & Cliffs: A Guide for Workforce Development Practitioners and Policymakers Serving Youth with Mental Health Needs,* Office of Disability Employment Policy Number #E-9-4-1-0070 (Washington, D.C.: March 2007).

[70] [70]SAMHSA has also developed as part of the Partnerships for Youth in Transition demonstration, an age-appropriate outcome measurement tool as well as a program fidelity instrument to assess how well programs are implemented. According to HHS, the existence of such standardized tools is a critical precursor to conducting randomized trails of the model.

[71] SAMHSA launched "What a Difference a Friend Makes," as part of the Mental Health Campaign for Mental Health Recovery, which is designed to encourage, educate, and inspire people between 18 and 25 to support their friends who are experiencing mental health problems.

[72] Job Corps, administered by Labor, is an education and job training program for at-risk youth age 16 through 24.

[73] Kessler, R., W. T. Chiu, L. Colpe, O. Demler, K. Merikangas, E. Walters, and P. Wang. "The Prevalence and Correlates of Serious Mental Illness (SMI) in the National Comorbidity Survey Replication (NCS-R)." In *Mental Health, United States, 2004,* ed. R.W. Manderscheid and Berry, J.T. DHHS Pub No. (SMA)-06-4195. Rockville, Maryland: Substance Abuse and Mental Health Services Administration, 2006.

[74] Respondents were determined to have a serious mental illness if they met any of the following criteria within the previous 12 months: made a serious suicide attempt; experienced a work disability or other substantial limitation because of a mental or substance disorder; or were diagnosed with bipolar I or II disorder, nonaffective psychosis, substance dependence with serious role impairment, impulse control disorder with repeated serious violence, or any disorder that resulted in 30 or more days functioning out of role in the year.

[75] We used weights specific to part 2 of the NCS-R for estimates of severity.

[76] According to the CPS, the population of 18-26--year-olds increased by about 7 percent from 2001 to 2006, from approximately 34.6 million to 37 million.

[77] The survey was administered in two parts. Part 1 contained a core diagnostic assessment while part 2 contained questions pertaining to specific behaviors, risk factors, and severity of mental illness. All respondents who met lifetime criteria for a mental illness in part 1 participated in part 2, as well as a probability subsample of those with no mental illness.

[78] Because the NCS-R employed a probability procedure based on random selections, the selected sample was only one of a large number of samples that might have been drawn. Since each sample could have provided different estimates, we express our confidence in the precision of the particular sample's results as a 95 percent confidence interval (e.g., plus or minus 12 percentage points). This is the interval that would contain the actual population value for 95 percent of the samples that could have been drawn. As a result, we are 95 percent confident that each of the confidence intervals in this report will include the true values in the study population.

[79] Mathematica Policy Research, Inc. developed these groupings as part of its evaluation of the Ticket to Work Program. Because we define "mental illness" to exclude mental disorders that constitute abnormalities in cognition or intellectual functioning, we excluded individuals whose primary disabling condition was listed as mental retardation, autistic disorder, other pervasive development disorders, organic mental disorders (chronic brain syndrome), or somatoform disorders. We also excluded eating and tic disorders and substance abuse disorders.

[80] In determining primary and secondary disabilities, we excluded SSI recipients who began receiving benefits as children and had not yet been redetermined by SSA under adult eligibility criteria. According to our analysis, this applied to about 32 percent of the total SSI population aged 18-26. DI recipients are not subject to the redetermination process

[81] Other state agencies that collaborated in the development of this program are the Office of Policy and Management and the Department of Mental Retardation.

[82] The levels of care are based on the young adults' clinical needs and are generally geared to help them develop increasing levels of independence and success in the community. Young adults receiving mental health services can access various levels of care during their recovery, depending on their clinical needs.

[83] Basic case management services consist of office-based and outreach visits on a monthly, biweekly, or weekly basis. The highly structured programs include: the specialized apartment program, designed for those that require staff in the apartment for nearly all day; group homes, which are congregate residential programs where individuals develop life skill, and specialized residential services programs with staff and supervision usually 24 hours a day seven days a week. A Connecticut mental health official told us that Connecticut primarily uses intensive case management, which is similar to the Assertive Community Treatment model, but does not meet all the criteria for Assertive Community Treatment, including having a psychiatrist available 24 hours a day seven days a week.

[84] See Davis, Maryann and Ann Vander Stoep. *The Transition to Adulthood Among Adolescents Who Have Serious Emotional Disturbance*, prepared for The National Resource Center on Homelessness and Mental Illness Policy Research Associates, Inc. Delmar, New York: under contract to the Center for Mental Health

Services, Substance Abuse and Mental Health Services Administration, April 1996; and Davis, Maryann. "Improving Youth Transitions Systems and Measuring Change." Presentation at the National Partnerships for Youth in Transition Forum, Center for Mental Health Services, Massachusetts: August 2005.

Index

R

S

Y